Retirement Activities: Embracing Life's New Chapter

Things to Do to Explore, Prosper, and Achieve Your Dreams Post-Retirement

Lorie Eubank

GTO Publishing Solutions, LLC.

CONTENTS

INTRODUCTION

Welcome to "Retirement Activities: Embracing Life's New Chapter" – your personal guidebook as you embark on one of life's most exciting adventures: retirement! If you're reading this, you're either on the cusp of retiring or have recently traded in your work shoes for a more comfortable pair. Whichever the case, give yourself a pat on the back. You've earned this moment!

Retirement is often pictured as an extended holiday, but let's be honest – it's so much more. It's a time brimming with potential, a chance to rediscover yourself, and an opportunity to craft a lifestyle that's as dynamic and fulfilling as any working period if not more. Think of this book as your friendly companion, guiding you through this vibrant journey.

We've packed these pages with ideas, stories, and practical tips to help you navigate this new phase with ease and enthusiasm. We cover everything from unraveling the emotional aspects of retiring to finding new hobbies, from financial planning to maintaining an active social life. But it's not just about the 'what' and 'how'; it's about the 'why.' Why embrace change? Why seek new passions? Why not just settle into a quiet life? The answer is simple: because this chapter of your life can be as enriching and exciting as you make it.

We'll look into the art of mastering the retirement lifestyle, exploring avenues you've never considered. Have you ever thought about learning a new language, starting a garden, or even joining a drum circle? How about volunteering in a way that leverages your lifetime of experience? There's a world of possibilities out there, and it's waiting for you.

So, whether you're excited, apprehensive, or a mix of both about this new chapter, rest assured, you're not alone. This book is here to inspire, support, and cheer you on. Let's turn these pages and begin this incredible journey together. Here's to exploring, prospering, and achieving your dreams in retirement. The adventure begins now!

Chapter 1: Embracing Change: A Fresh Look at Retirement

"Don't simply retire from something; have something to retire to." - Harry Emerson Fosdick

1.1 Debunking Common Retirement Misconceptions

Let's start with the first misconception:

Myth: Retirement means slowing down

Many people think that retirement is a time to slow down, a period of declining energy and activity. But this couldn't be further from the truth. Retirement is not synonymous with inactivity. In fact, it's quite the opposite. It's a time to engage in activities that you love and make you feel alive. It's a time to be active, not in the sense of rushing to and from work or meeting deadlines, but in terms of engaging in stimulating activities, be it physical, mental, or social.

Myth: You'll be bored without work

Work provides structure to our lives, and it's natural to wonder what will fill our days when it's no longer part of our routine. But retirement doesn't mean the end of productivity or purpose. Think about it. How often have you said, "I wish I had more time for..."? Well, retirement provides that time. It's a chance to fill your days with activities that bring you joy, satisfaction, and a sense of accomplishment.

Myth: It's too late to start new hobbies

I've met several people who think that new hobbies are for the younger generation and it's too late for them to start something new. But age should never be a barrier to learning. Many retirees discover new hobbies and passions during their retirement years. Think about it. You have a wealth of life experience to draw from, patience that comes with age, and the freedom of time. These are the perfect ingredients for brewing a new hobby.

Watching different artists online inspired me to try various forms of painting, from paint pouring to traditional acrylic painting to watercolors and lettering (yes, that is an art form). I even tried my hand at following Bob Ross videos. All in the name of dreaming of what I could do when I don't have a 9 to 5 job to report to every day.

So, whether it's learning to play a musical instrument, starting a book club, or even going back to school, retirement is the perfect time to explore these opportunities. And when you are looking for opportunities and new things to try, check out your local senior center. The activities they plan can also help you to meet others who are finding their way into retirement or have been there a while.

Retirement is like a blank canvas, and you hold the brush. It's an opportunity to paint a picture of life as you want it to be, free from the constraints of a 9 to 5 job. It's a time to explore, to learn, and to grow. So, lace up those running shoes, pick up that paintbrush, or dust off that guitar. Your retirement is waiting for you to make it truly golden.

1.2 Understanding the Emotional Rollercoaster of Retirement

Welcome to the exhilarating world of retirement—a chapter in your life where emotions take center stage. Beyond the spreadsheets and retirement calculators, there's a rich tapestry of feelings that often accompany this transition. So, let's dive deep into the emotional rollercoaster that is retirement because understanding these sentiments is the key to unlocking a fulfilling and meaningful post-career life.

As you prepare to bid adieu to the 9-to-5 routine, you may find yourself on an emotional journey that rivals any theme park thrill ride. It starts with the excitement of newfound freedom—the thrill of waking up without an alarm clock, the liberation of not having to endure rush-hour traffic, and the sheer joy of reclaiming your time. This newfound freedom is like stepping into a world where every day is a Saturday, and the possibilities are endless.

Yet, along with this excitement, there may be an undercurrent of uncertainty. Change, even when it's desired, can be a bit daunting. You might question if you're making the right choice, wonder if you'll miss the structure of work, or worry about how your identity might shift when you're no longer defined by your career. These are natural concerns, and acknowledging them is the first step in navigating this emotional terrain.

On this rollercoaster, you'll also experience moments of nostalgia. Memories of the workplace—the camaraderie, the challenges, the achievements—can evoke bittersweet feelings. It's perfectly normal to miss the people and the routines that have been a part of your life for so long.

But here's the exhilarating twist: as you journey through this emotional landscape, you'll discover newfound passions, interests, and opportunities that you never had the time to explore before. Retirement offers a canvas for reinvention, a chance to rediscover who you are and what truly makes your heart sing. It's a time to embrace change, celebrate the wisdom of your years, and to savor the freedom of pursuing your own dreams and desires.

So, dear reader, as we embark on this adventure together, remember that understanding the emotional rollercoaster of retirement is like knowing the twists and turns of a thrilling ride. It's all part of the journey, and with each loop, you'll gain a deeper appreciation for the exhilarating path ahead. Get ready to embrace change, and let's explore the myriad possibilities of your retirement with excitement, optimism, and a heart open to new adventures.

1.3 Embracing Change: The Path to a Fulfilling Retirement

The Change is not merely an occasional guest in the realm of retirement; it's the heartbeat that keeps this new chapter alive and thriving. It's a force that propels you forward, a dynamic companion on this exhilarating journey. In this section, we're going to delve deeper into the idea that embracing change is the key to unlocking a retirement that is brimming with purpose, fulfillment, and unending adventures. So, put on your explorer's hat, for we are about to embark on a journey of transformation and growth—a path that promises to redefine the way you look at retirement.

Retirement is, in many ways, a grand opportunity for reinvention. It's a time to reinvent yourself, your goals, and your aspirations. It's a chance to step boldly into the unknown and declare, "This is my time." Imagine your life as a canvas and retirement as the moment when you pick up the brush to paint the masterpiece of your dreams. Embracing change means surrendering to the artistic process of self-discovery and renewal.

As you transition from the structured world of work to the freedom of retirement, it's perfectly natural to feel a bit off balance. After all, you're navigating uncharted waters. But it's precisely in these moments of uncertainty that the magic happens. You begin to explore new interests, hobbies, and passions that you may have set aside during your working years. You have the time and space to dive into activities that bring you joy and fulfillment. Whether it's learning to play a musical instrument, taking up painting, joining a local theater group, or even starting a new career, retirement grants you the license to pursue your passions with gusto.

Moreover, embracing change in retirement isn't just about reinventing yourself; it's about evolving your relationships and expanding your horizons. You have the opportunity to connect with new people who share your interests and passions, forming bonds that can enrich your life in unexpected ways. Volunteering, joining clubs, or participating in community events can open doors to meaningful connections and experiences you never thought possible.

It's important to recognize that change doesn't have to be monumental to be transformative. Even small shifts in your daily routines and mindset can lead to significant personal growth and a heightened sense of fulfillment. Embracing change is about being adaptable, curious, and open to new experiences.

As you venture on this path to a fulfilling retirement, remember that change is not something to be feared but rather celebrated. It's the catalyst for your personal growth, the gateway to exciting adventures, and the roadmap to discovering new dimensions of joy and purpose. Embrace the ever-evolving landscape of your post-career life with enthusiasm, and let change be the fuel that propels you toward a retirement that is nothing short of extraordinary.

1.4 Finding New Purpose: The Joy of Post-Retirement Passions

Ah, retirement—a chapter where the past meets the future, and the seeds of your long-held dreams finally have the chance to flourish. It's a phase of life that invites you to step into your passions, embrace your desires, and rekindle the fires of purpose that may have dimmed during your working years. In this section, we're going to explore the exhilarating world of discovering and nurturing those passions, reigniting your sense of purpose, and infusing your retirement with newfound vitality. So, get ready to embark on a journey of self-discovery that will unveil the joys of post-retirement passions.

For many of us, our working lives often leave little room to indulge in our interests and hobbies fully. The demands of our careers can lead us to set aside those dreams and activities that truly light our souls on fire. But retirement changes the game entirely. It's like being handed a golden ticket to explore the passions that have been simmering on the back burner for far too long.

So, what is it that makes your heart race with excitement? Is it painting, gardening, playing a musical instrument, or perhaps volunteering for a cause you're passionate about? Retirement offers you the luxury of time to dive headfirst into these pursuits and rediscover the boundless joy they bring. You have the opportunity to become the artist you've always wanted to be, cultivate the garden of your dreams, or master that musical instrument that has beckoned you for years. The possibilities are as vast as your imagination.

Moreover, embracing post-retirement passions is not only about indulging in activities you love but also about cultivating a deeper sense of purpose. When you pursue what truly moves you, you tap into a wellspring of enthusiasm and motivation. You'll find that your days are no longer about just passing the time but about creating a life that resonates with authenticity and meaning.

Exploring new passions in retirement can also lead to unexpected adventures and connections. You may join clubs or groups centered around your interests, providing you with opportunities to meet like-minded individuals who share your zeal. These connections can bring a sense of belonging and camaraderie, providing a fulfilling social life that extends beyond the workplace.

In retirement, you have the incredible gift of time, and it's up to you how you choose to spend it. By diving into your passions and rediscovering your sense of purpose, you breathe new life into your post-career years. It's not just about growing older; it's about growing wiser, more passionate, and more in tune with the things that truly matter to you.

So, as you explore the joy of post-retirement passions, remember that retirement is not an endpoint but a remarkable new beginning. It's a chance to reconnect with your authentic self, reignite your sense of purpose, and infuse each day with vitality and enthusiasm. Your passions are waiting to be rediscovered, and retirement is the perfect time to set them free. Embrace this extraordinary journey, and let your heart lead you to a retirement filled with joy and fulfillment.

Chapter 2: Journey to Self: Discovering Your Retirement Identity

> *"Retirement is when you stop living at work and start working at living." - Unknown*

Picture yourself standing before a grand buffet, a culinary spread that spans the horizon. The dishes are as diverse as they are numerous, a smorgasbord of flavors, textures, and aromas. And the best part? You're free to pick and choose whatever catches your fancy. No restrictions, no rules, just a world of delicious choices waiting for you to savor. That, my dear friend, is much like retirement, an expansive buffet of life where you get to pick and choose what defines or excites you in this new phase.

The transition from a full-time career to retirement often prompts a crucial question – Who am I now? This question, though simple, carries profound implications. It's about understanding what makes you, YOU, outside the context of a job title or professional role. It's about reflecting on your personal values, identifying your strengths and talents, and recognizing your interests. Together, these elements form the core of your identity in retirement, the unique blend that makes you who you are.

2.1 Who Am I Now? Finding Your Identity Post-Retirement

Reflecting on Personal Values

Values are the compass that guides our actions, the underlying principles that shape our attitudes and behaviors. They are the bedrock of our character, the essence of who we are. As you step into retirement, it's essential to reflect on your values and understand how they can shape your retirement life.

Consider this: Grab a notebook and create a list of values that resonate with you. Honesty, compassion, courage, humor, respect, creativity, family, freedom, health, peace, wisdom – the list can be as long as you want it to be. Now, from this list, pick the top five values that resonate with you the most. These are your core values, the guiding principles that you want to base your retirement life on.

For instance, if creativity is one of your core values, you might want to fill your retirement days with activities that stimulate your creative side, like painting, writing, or playing a musical instrument. If health is a core value, regular exercise, a balanced diet, and routine health check-ups could be a vital part of your retirement routine.

Reflecting on personal values isn't just about understanding what's important to you. It's also about aligning your retirement life with these values to create a fulfilling and meaningful existence.

Identifying Strengths and Talents

Remember the joy of childhood when you could spend hours doing something simply because you were good at it and enjoyed it? Maybe you were great at solving puzzles, or perhaps you could play a musical instrument with ease. These are your strengths and talents, and they can play a significant role in shaping your retirement identity.

Your strengths are those skills that you are naturally good at. It could be anything from gardening to cooking, from painting to writing. Talents, on the other hand, are those inherent abilities that you have, like a knack for numbers, a flair for languages, or a natural rhythm that makes you a great dancer.

Identifying your strengths and talents can open up a world of possibilities for your retirement life. It can help you choose activities that you're likely to enjoy and excel at. For example, if you're naturally good with numbers, you might enjoy taking up Sudoku or other number puzzles. If you have a talent for languages, learning a new language could be an exciting venture for you.

Recognizing Personal Interests

In the hustle and bustle of working life, personal interests often take a backseat. But in retirement, these interests can take center stage. Do you love reading? Join a book club or set a reading challenge for yourself. Are you fascinated by history? Visit museums, watch documentaries, or even take up a history course.

Your personal interests can form the foundation of your retirement activities. They can fill your days with joy, satisfaction, and a sense of fulfillment. Moreover, pursuing your interests can also lead to new social connections. Joining clubs or groups that share your interests can provide a sense of belonging and community, adding a social dimension to your retirement life.

So, as you stand before the grand buffet of retirement, take your time to explore, to taste, and savor. Reflect on your values, recognize your strengths and talents, and reignite your personal interests. These are the ingredients that will spice up your retirement life, adding richness, flavor, and a sense of fulfillment to your golden years. Remember, this is your buffet, your retirement, and your life. Make it count!

2.2 Hobbies and Interests: The Building Blocks of Your New Life

Gardening

Imagine stepping outside to a symphony of colors and fragrances. Butterflies flit about, birds chirp from the trees, and amidst it all, you stand, trowel in hand, ready for a day of gardening. From planting seeds to seeing them sprout and bloom, gardening is a pastime that's not just enjoyable but also deeply rewarding.

Each plant, each flower, and each herb you grow is a testament to your patience and care. And the best part? Gardening isn't just about colorful flower beds or lush green lawns. It can also be about growing your own food. Imagine the joy of making a salad with tomatoes from your garden or seasoning your pasta with homegrown herbs. Gardening offers a sense of accomplishment and lets you reap the literal fruits of your labor.

Painting

A blank canvas, a palette of colors, and an artist's brush - that's all you need to embark on a journey of creativity and self-expression. Painting is a hobby that lets you capture the world as you see it or even as you imagine it. It's a form of expression that transcends language and speaks directly to the heart.

Whether you choose to paint landscapes, portraits, or abstract art, each stroke of your brush is a reflection of your thoughts, feelings, and creativity. And remember, painting isn't about creating a masterpiece every time. It's about enjoying the process, about the peace and tranquility that comes from focusing on your canvas and letting your creativity flow.

Bird Watching

The world outside your window is full of life, and bird-watching is a fantastic way to connect with nature's winged wonders. Each bird, with its distinct colors, patterns, and songs, is a marvel to behold. Whether you're spotting robins in your backyard or seeking out rare species in a nature reserve, bird watching is a hobby that's as exciting as it is enriching.

Armed with a pair of binoculars and a bird guide, you can spend hours observing these delightful creatures, learning about their habits and behaviors. Plus, bird watching encourages you to spend time outdoors, in the lap of nature, which is always a good thing.

Cooking

The kitchen is more than just a space for preparing meals. It's a playground for flavor, a canvas for culinary creativity. Cooking as a hobby is not just about feeding the body but also about nourishing the soul. It's about the joy of creating something delicious and sharing it with others.

Retirement offers the perfect opportunity to explore the world of cooking. Try out new recipes, experiment with exotic ingredients, or even master your family's traditional dishes. Every meal you prepare is a celebration of taste, a testament to your culinary skills, and an expression of your love for good food.

Photography

In the age of smartphones, everyone can be a photographer. But photography as a hobby is more than just snapping pictures. It's about capturing moments, emotions, and the beauty of the world around us.

With a camera in hand, you start to see the world differently. You notice the play of light and shadow, the vibrancy of colors, and the beauty in everyday scenes. Each photo you take is a freeze-frame of a moment in time, a visual narrative that tells a story. Whether you prefer capturing landscapes, portraits, wildlife, or abstract images, photography is a hobby that combines creativity, observation, and technical skills.

In the grand buffet of retirement, these hobbies and interests are just a few of the many dishes you can choose from. They're not just ways to pass the time but also opportunities for learning, creativity, and personal growth. There are online courses available for all of these hobby options, and you can get discounts for 50-80% off through services like Groupon. Depending on the timing, you could take a class at your local community college to not only deepen your understanding of the topic but also enjoy the community experience.

So, go ahead, don your gardening gloves, pick up your paintbrush, grab your binoculars, put on your chef's hat, or reach for your camera. Your retirement is waiting for you to add your unique flavor to it.

2.3 The Power of Passion: Pursuing What You Love

Imagine sitting at your desk, a blank page on your computer screen waiting to be filled with words. You let your mind wander, your fingers hover over the keyboard, and then, like a dam breaking, the words start to flow. Characters, dialogues, and scenes all come to life as you weave a narrative that's uniquely yours. This is the power of writing, the power to create worlds and characters that exist only in your imagination and through your words, on the page.

Writing a Novel

Writing a novel is a labor of love, a test of perseverance, and a testament to the power of creativity. It's a way to tell stories, express your thoughts, and explore the depths of human emotions. Whether it's a thrilling mystery, a heartwarming romance, or a thought-provoking piece of literary fiction, every novel you write is a piece of your heart served on a platter of words.

In retirement, you have the luxury of time and the freedom of imagination to pen down your novel. You can write at your own pace without the pressure of deadlines. Whether you choose to publish your work or keep it as a personal treasure, the joy of writing a novel is in the journey, in seeing your ideas take shape and come to life.

If a novel seems too large to tackle, a memoir is a great place to start. Capture the memories of your life, where you grew up, school memories, places you lived, and places you traveled to. This is a great way to pass down family history to the next generations.

Starting a Small Business

Perhaps you've always dreamed of being your own boss or of starting a venture that reflects your values and interests. Retirement could be the perfect time to turn this dream into reality. Starting a small business in retirement not only provides an avenue for income but also offers a sense of purpose and fulfillment.

It could be a bakery churning out delicious treats for the local community. Or a gardening service, helping others create their own little patch of green. It might even be an online store selling handmade fishing lures or vintage collectibles. The key is to choose a business idea that aligns with your interests, skills, and passions.

Remember, starting a business doesn't mean plunging into stressful work schedules again. The beauty of a retirement business is that you call the shots. You set your hours, you choose the projects, and you decide how you want to grow your business. It's a chance to create something that's truly yours, something that reflects your passion and dedication.

Learning a Musical Instrument

Picture this: it's a quiet afternoon; you're sitting in your favorite armchair, a guitar in your hands and a melody in your heart. As your fingers strum the strings, the notes fill the room, creating a symphony that's as soothing as it is uplifting. This is the beauty of music, the power it holds to stir emotions and touch souls.

Learning a musical instrument in retirement is like opening a new window to the world. It's not just about mastering the notes but also about understanding the rhythm, the melody, and the emotion that music conveys. Whether it's a guitar, a piano, a violin, or even your voice, every instrument has a unique sound, a unique flavor that adds to the symphony of life.

Moreover, learning a musical instrument is also a great way to keep your mind sharp and active. It challenges your memory, coordination, and concentration skills. And let's not forget the joy of playing your favorite tune, of creating music that resonates with your soul.

Retirement is a time to follow your passions, to do what you love, and to explore new avenues of self-expression. So, go ahead, write that novel, start that business, or learn that musical instrument. Let your passion guide your retirement journey; let it add color, excitement, and fulfillment to your golden years. After all, retirement is not the end of the road, but the beginning of a new, exciting path, a path paved with opportunities, possibilities, and, most importantly, the power of passion.

2.4 Opportunities for Self-Discovery

Solo Travel

Picture this: you've just landed in a city you've never been to before. The language is different, the food is exotic, and the culture is unique. You feel a mix of excitement, curiosity, and maybe even a little bit of apprehension. Welcome to the world of solo travel – an adventure that's all about discovery, exploration, and personal growth.

Traveling solo offers a unique opportunity for self-discovery. It's a chance to step out of your comfort zone, to face challenges head-on, and to learn about yourself in ways you never imagined. From navigating foreign cities to trying new cuisines, every experience shapes you, molds you, and adds to your story.

Solo travel also gives you the freedom to set your own pace, and to follow your own itinerary. You can spend hours exploring a museum, relax in a city park, or simply sit at a sidewalk café and watch the world go by. The choice is yours, and the journey is yours alone.

Joining a Book Club

Imagine sitting in a cozy living room, a cup of tea in your hand, and a group of fellow book lovers around you. The air is filled with animated discussions, varying perspectives, and shared laughter. This is what joining a book club is all about – a community of readers who share your passion for literature and offer a platform for intellectual stimulation and social interaction.

Being part of a book club not only broadens your reading horizons but also provides an opportunity for self-discovery.

As you discuss different books, share your interpretations, and listen to others' viewpoints, you gain insights into your own thought processes, beliefs, and attitudes.

A book club offers more than just a monthly meeting. It's a circle of friends, a support system, and a space for intellectual and emotional growth. So, pick up that novel, dive into its pages, and get ready to share, discuss, and discover.

Attending Workshops

Remember the thrill of the first day of school? The excitement of learning something new, the anticipation of new challenges, and the joy of expanding your knowledge. Attending workshops in retirement can bring back that same thrill, that same joy of learning.

Workshops offer a hands-on, interactive approach to learning. Whether it's a cooking class, a photography workshop, or a writing seminar, you get the chance to learn from experts, practice your skills, and receive immediate feedback.

Each workshop is a step towards self-improvement, a step towards honing your talents and exploring your interests. It's a chance to challenge yourself, to push your boundaries, and to discover your potential. So, sign up for that workshop, learn that new skill, and let the joy of learning fuel your retirement days.

Retirement is an exciting phase of life filled with countless opportunities for self-discovery. It's a time to explore, to learn, and to grow as an individual. Whether you're traversing foreign cities, discussing literature with fellow book lovers, or learning a new skill in a workshop, each experience shapes you, molds you, and adds to your retirement story. So, go ahead, seize these opportunities, and let the adventure of self-discovery begin.

As we conclude, remember that retirement is your time, a time to focus on yourself. You've spent a lifetime working, taking care of others, and fulfilling responsibilities. Now, it's your turn to enjoy, explore, and experience. The world is your oyster, and retirement is your pearl. Cherish it, embrace it, and make the most of it. Now, let's move forward to the next exciting part of this book.

Chapter 3: Nurturing Your Mind and Soul

"*Retire from work, but not from life.*" - *M.K. Soni*

Imagine a sunny morning, the birds chirping, the aroma of your favorite coffee filling the air. You're sitting on the porch, a notebook in hand, and you're writing down three things you're grateful for. This simple act, this moment of gratitude, has the power to shift your perspective, brighten your day, to change your life. Welcome to Chapter 3, where we explore the power of positivity, the joy of lifelong learning, and the importance of keeping your mind engaged in retirement.

3.1 Embracing Positivity: A New Mindset for Retirement

Practicing Gratitude

Gratitude is like a beacon of light that can illuminate even the darkest corners of our minds. It's about focusing on what's good in our lives, acknowledging our blessings, and expressing appreciation. It's the act of counting our blessings rather than dwelling on what's lacking.

How can you practice gratitude in retirement? It's as simple as keeping a gratitude journal. Each morning, jot down three things you're grateful for. It could be something as simple as a good night's sleep, a call from an old friend, or the smell of fresh bread from your kitchen.

When you practice gratitude regularly, you tend to focus more on the positive aspects of your life. This shift in focus can significantly enhance your happiness, reduce stress, and improve your overall well-being.

Focusing on the Present

Often, we're so caught up in the memories of the past or the worries of the future that we forget to live in the present. But the present moment is where life happens. It's where joy resides, where peace prevails. It is like opening a present full of opportunities for you to do what inspires you and makes you happy. But not just happy; it is an opportunity to find purpose in the day that you don't want to miss out on.

Retirement offers the freedom to truly live in the present. Without the stress of work deadlines or the hustle of a busy career, you can fully immerse yourself in the 'now.'

Take a walk in the park and notice the beauty around you - the rustling leaves, the blooming flowers, the children playing. Sit quietly in your favorite armchair with a good book and let yourself be drawn into the story. Attend a pottery class and let your hands and mind work in harmony as you shape the clay.

Focusing on the present allows you to experience life in its fullness, one moment at a time. It's not about forgetting the past or ignoring the future; it's about giving your undivided attention to the 'now' and savoring it.

Celebrating Small Victories

In the race of life, we often overlook the small victories, waiting for the big wins to celebrate. But retirement is a time to change this mindset. It's a time to celebrate every victory, no matter how small.

Finished reading a book? That's a win. Tried a new recipe, and it turned out great. That's a win. You walked an extra mile more than usual. That's a win. Every small achievement adds to your self-confidence, self-esteem, and sense of accomplishment.

So, go ahead, and celebrate your small victories. It could be a pat on your back, a happy dance, or a treat from your favorite bakery. Each celebration, however small, adds a dash of joy to your retirement life and motivates you to keep going.

Positivity in retirement isn't about turning a blind eye to the challenges or difficulties. It's about choosing to focus on the bright side to nurture a mindset that's geared toward happiness, gratitude, and contentment. It's about practicing gratitude, living in the present, and celebrating small victories. This positive mindset can be your greatest ally in making your retirement a truly golden phase of life.

3.2 Mindfulness and Meditation: Tools for Mental Peace

In the stillness of the early morning, even before the first light of dawn breaks, there's a serene calmness, a quiet that's both soothing and revitalizing. Imagine yourself in this quietude, sitting comfortably, your eyes closed, your mind alert yet relaxed. This is the beginning of a mindfulness practice, a journey towards inner peace and mental well-being.

Guided Meditation

Meditation might seem daunting at first, especially if you're new to the practice. Fear not, for guided meditation is a perfect starting point. It's akin to having a personal guide accompanying you on a hike, leading the way, and ensuring you're on the right path.

In guided meditation, a narrator or teacher provides step-by-step instructions, leading you through the process. These instructions could be in the form of a recorded audio track, a video, or even a live session. All you need to do is find a quiet, comfortable spot, put on your headphones, and allow the guide to lead you into a state of deep relaxation and awareness.

The beauty of guided meditation is its versatility. You can choose from a plethora of themes, such as stress relief, self-love, or even sleep enhancement. Start with just a few minutes each day and gradually increase the duration as you become more comfortable with the practice.

Yoga

Imagine yourself standing tall, your feet firmly planted on the ground, your arms reaching up towards the sky. This is the mountain pose, a simple yet powerful yoga pose that embodies strength and stability. It's also a metaphor for what yoga can do for your mind – grounding you in the present and helping you reach for a state of calm and tranquility.

Yoga is more than just a physical exercise; it's a holistic practice that combines postures, breath control, and meditation. It's about creating a balance between the body, mind, and spirit. A typical yoga session includes a series of postures or 'asanas,' breathing exercises or 'pranayama,' and a period of meditation or relaxation.

Yoga, with its emphasis on mindful movements and conscious breathing, is a perfect complement to your retirement lifestyle. It not only helps maintain physical flexibility but also promotes mental peace and mindfulness. And the best part? You don't need to be super flexible or incredibly fit to practice yoga. There are styles and postures to suit every fitness level.

I will make one recommendation on the area of resources for Yoga. I have really enjoyed DDPY yoga as the creator of the program used Yoga as a tool in recovering from an injury. He offers Bed Flex exercises, chair yoga, and beginner through advanced. You can work at your own level. The program is available on DVD or an app that you can take with you on the go. I used the app and took it on a cruise when I celebrated my 50th birthday, and I use the DVDs at home.

There are also a number of books, audiobooks, and DVDs available, as well as community centers that offer great teachings on how to use Yoga as a form of everyday exercise to ensure you keep your body flexible and moving. If you don't like the first resource, look at other options. I started yoga in the gym in my 30s as a follow-up class for strength training. When I gave up my gym membership, I tried a few different DVDs, I even used the Wii Fit with the balance board to add some variety. Find what works for you and have fun with it.

So no matter what option you choose, roll out that yoga mat and experience the harmony of mind, body, and breath.

Deep Breathing Exercises

Picture a serene lake, its surface calm and undisturbed. Now, imagine a pebble being dropped into the lake. It creates ripples that spread across the surface, disturbing the calm waters. Stress and anxiety are like those pebbles, creating ripples in the calm lake of your mind. Deep breathing exercises can be your shield against these ripples, helping maintain the tranquility of your mind.

Deep breathing, also known as diaphragmatic breathing, involves breathing deeply into your lungs by engaging your diaphragm. This type of breathing slows your heartbeat, lowers or stabilizes blood pressure, and can help you relax.

Here's a simple deep breathing exercise you can try: Sit comfortably, close your eyes, and take a slow, deep breath in through your nose. Try to fill your lungs with air, letting your belly expand as you breathe in. Hold your breath for a few seconds and then exhale slowly through your mouth, letting your belly fall. Repeat this process for a few minutes, focusing on your breath as you inhale and exhale.

Deep breathing exercises can be your go-to tool for instant relaxation, a handy shield against the stressors of life. Whether you're feeling anxious about a doctor's appointment or struggling to fall asleep, a few minutes of deep breathing can help calm your mind and relax your body.

In the grand tapestry of retirement, mindfulness and meditation are the threads that can add a sense of calm and tranquility. They're tools to help you navigate the ebbs and flows of life with grace and poise. So, embrace these practices, weave them into your daily routine, and experience the transformation they bring to your retirement life.

3.3 Lifelong Learning: The Joy of New Knowledge

Consider a moment when you discovered something new. Recall that spark of interest, the curiosity it ignited, and the satisfaction that came with understanding. That, my dear friend, is the joy of learning. And guess what? Retirement is the perfect time to fan the flames of this joy, to feed your curiosity, and to immerse yourself in the river of knowledge.

Online Courses

In today's digital age, learning has no boundaries. From the comfort of your living room, you can explore the mysteries of the universe, understand the intricacies of the human brain, or dive into the history of ancient civilizations. This is the power of online courses - a vast ocean of knowledge at your fingertips.

Online platforms like Coursera, edX, and Khan Academy offer courses on a wide array of subjects. Interested in photography?

There's a course for that. Fascinated by astronomy? There's a course for that too. The best part? You can learn at your own pace. Pause, rewind, rewatch - you control your learning journey.

Taking an online course isn't just about gaining knowledge. It's also about challenging your mind and keeping it sharp and active. It's about the thrill of understanding complex concepts, the satisfaction of completing assignments, and the pride of earning a certificate. It's your personal victory, a testament to the power of lifelong learning.

Local Community Classes

While online learning offers convenience and flexibility, local community classes offer something equally valuable - social interaction. Picture this: you're in a room full of like-minded individuals, all there to learn, just like you. The air buzzes with excitement, curiosity, and the shared joy of learning.

Community colleges, adult education centers, and even local libraries often offer a variety of classes for seniors. These could range from painting and pottery to computer skills and foreign languages. Some classes might even focus on topics of particular interest to retirees, like financial planning or health and wellness.

Joining a community class is a perfect blend of learning and socializing. It's an opportunity to meet new people, to engage in stimulating discussions, and to learn in a supportive and interactive environment. So, go ahead, and check out the classes offered in your local community. Sign up for something that piques your interest and get ready for a rewarding and enriching experience.

Reading Groups

Remember the joy of getting lost in a good book, of traveling to far-off places, meeting fascinating characters, and living a thousand lives, all within the pages of a novel? Now, imagine sharing this joy with others, discussing plot twists, dissecting characters, and diving deeper into the story. Welcome to reading groups, your passport to a world of literary exploration.

Reading groups, or book clubs, bring together people who share a love for books. It could be a group of friends who meet monthly at each other's homes or a community-wide group coordinated by the local library. Some groups focus on specific genres like mystery or historical fiction, while others are more eclectic.

Joining a reading group can add a new dimension to your reading experience. It's not just about the books but also about the discussions, the diverse perspectives, and the shared love for literature. It's about discovering new authors, genres, and themes. It's about the joy of sharing a good book and the excitement of diving into a new one.

Retirement offers the gift of time, a gift that you can use to learn, explore, to satisfy your curiosity. As you journey through this phase of life, let the joy of learning be your companion. Let it ignite your curiosity, stimulate your mind, and enrich your life. Whether through online courses, community classes, or reading groups, embrace the opportunities for lifelong learning that retirement brings. After all, every day is a chance to learn something new, to add a new chapter to your book of life.

3.4 Mental Exercises: Keeping Your Brain Engaged

Remember those lazy Sunday afternoons? You're lounging on your favorite chair, a steaming cup of tea by your side and a crossword puzzle in front of you. As your mind sifts through the clues, connecting the dots, filling in the blanks, there's a sense of anticipation, a spark of excitement. This is more than just a way to pass the time; it's a mental exercise, a workout for your brain.

Crossword Puzzles

Crossword puzzles are like a treasure hunt for words. Each clue leads you to a word, and each word fits into the puzzle, creating a network of interconnected letters. From simple wordplay to cryptic clues, crossword puzzles come in various levels of complexity, catering to a wide range of word enthusiasts.

Crossword puzzles not only improve your vocabulary but also enhance your problem-solving skills. They require you to think critically, to make connections, and to recall information. In essence, they give your brain a workout, helping keep it sharp and agile.

So grab a crossword puzzle, get your thinking cap on, and let the word hunt begin. Whether you complete the puzzle or not, the joy lies in the process, in the thrill of the hunt, and in the satisfaction of finding the right word.

Memory Games

Memory games are a fun and interactive way to test and improve your recall. They stimulate your brain, challenge your memory, and are a great way to pass the time. From classic games like 'Concentration' to modern apps that you can play on your phone or tablet, memory games come in all shapes and sizes.

Playing memory games regularly can help enhance your short-term memory, improve your concentration, and even delay the onset of memory-related conditions. They keep your mind engaged and active, and, most importantly, they're enjoyable.

So, whether it's matching pairs of cards, remembering a sequence of numbers, or recalling objects in a picture, memory games offer an exciting and beneficial way to keep your brain in top shape. Ready for a round of memory challenges? Game on!

Learning a New Language

Imagine being able to converse with locals on your next trip to Spain, understanding the lyrics of your favorite Italian song, or even reading a French novel in its original language. Learning a new language opens up a world of possibilities. It's like being handed a key to a new world, a world that was always there but one that you can now explore more deeply.

But that's not all. Learning a new language is also a fantastic mental exercise. It improves your memory, enhances your listening skills, and even boosts your cognitive abilities. It requires you to understand new grammar rules, to expand your vocabulary, and to practice pronunciation. In other words, it offers a full package of mental workouts.

So, pick a language that intrigues you, sign up for a course, or download a language learning app, and get started on this exciting linguistic adventure. Who knows? You might just discover a hidden talent for languages.

In conclusion, engaging your mind is just as crucial in retirement as keeping your body active. It's about maintaining your cognitive abilities, about keeping your brain cells buzzing with activity. It's about the joy of solving a crossword puzzle, the thrill of winning a memory game, and the satisfaction of learning a new language. These mental exercises are more than just hobbies; they're a way to keep your brain fit and healthy. So, devote some time each day to these activities, challenge your mind, and enjoy the benefits they bring to your retirement life.

Life in retirement is a beautiful blend of relaxation and stimulation. It's about nurturing your mind and body. It's about embracing positivity, finding inner peace, and keeping your mind sharp and active. Whether through mindfulness practices, lifelong learning, or mental exercises, retirement offers countless opportunities to enrich your life. So, seize these opportunities, enrich your retirement life, and remember that the real joy lies in the journey, not the destination. Now, let's move forward to the next exciting chapter in this book.

Chapter 4: Staying Physically Active and Healthy

"For many, retirement is a time for personal growth, which becomes the path to greater freedom." –Robert Delamontague

Do you enjoy a beautiful, vintage car - let's say, a 1966 Ford Mustang? Now, imagine the car has been kept in pristine condition, its engine regularly serviced, its body polished to a high shine, and the interior meticulously cleaned. Even after decades, the car runs smoothly, its performance uncompromised. Why? Because it's been well cared for and maintained regularly. Your body, dear friends, is not much different. As we age, regular 'maintenance' becomes crucial to keep our 'machinery' running smoothly. That's why focusing on physical health in retirement is of utmost importance.

In this chapter, we'll be exploring the significance of physical health in retirement, guiding you through the steps to ensure you're firing on all cylinders, running as smoothly as that classic Mustang. Let's get started, shall we?

4.1 The Importance of Physical Health in Retirement

Your health is your wealth - it's not just a catchy phrase; it's a fundamental truth. As we journey into retirement, maintaining physical health becomes even more crucial. It's the foundation upon which we build our retirement activities, our zest for life, and our well-being. Let's break down the key components of maintaining physical health in retirement.

Regular Check-ups

Consider regular medical check-ups as 'routine servicing' for your body. Just as a car needs regular oil changes and tire rotations, our bodies need consistent medical evaluations. Regular check-ups can help detect potential health issues before they become severe problems.

These check-ups should include routine screenings recommended for your age and gender, such as blood pressure measurements, cholesterol level checks, cancer screenings, and eye and dental exams, among others. Regular check-ups provide an opportunity to update vaccinations and discuss any health concerns or changes you might have noticed with your doctor.

In addition to these, it's important to have regular medication reviews. If you're on long-term medication, this review can help assess whether the medication is still necessary or if the dosage needs adjustment. It's a good practice to keep a list of all the medications you're currently on, including any over-the-counter supplements or remedies, to discuss with your healthcare provider.

Balanced Diet

Think of food as the fuel that powers your body. Just as you would only want to put the best quality fuel in your prized Mustang, feeding your body with high-quality, nutritious food is critical.

A balanced diet is one that gives your body the nutrients it needs to function correctly. It's not about strict dietary limitations or depriving yourself of the foods you love. It's about feeling great, having more energy, and stabilizing your mood.

Aim to fill your plate with a rainbow of foods - the more colorful, the better. Fruits and vegetables should take up half of your plate. They are high in vitamins, minerals, and fiber but low in calories.

Lean proteins like fish, poultry, beans, and nuts are essential for maintaining muscle mass, something that tends to decrease as we age. Include whole grains like oats, brown rice, and whole grain bread or pasta for your dose of fiber and essential nutrients.

Remember, it's not just about what you eat, but also how much. Pay attention to portion sizes to avoid overeating. Listening to your body's hunger and fullness cues can help you maintain a healthy weight.

Adequate Sleep

Just as a car needs to be turned off and parked to function optimally, your body needs sleep to repair and rejuvenate itself. Sleep plays a vital role in physical health. It's during sleep that the body is hard at work repairing heart and blood vessels, maintaining a balance of hormones, and enhancing learning and memory function.

Most adults need 7 to 8 hours of good quality sleep per night. Establishing a regular sleep schedule, creating a restful environment, and making healthy lifestyle choices can significantly improve the quality of your sleep.

To sum up, maintaining physical health in retirement is about regular 'servicing' through medical check-ups, fueling your body with a balanced diet, and ensuring your body gets the rest it needs through adequate sleep. Just like that vintage Mustang, with regular care and maintenance, you can ensure that your 'engine' keeps running smoothly throughout your retirement years.

Let's pause here for a moment. Take a deep breath, reflect on the importance of physical health, and make a commitment to yourself to make it a priority in your retirement life. Remember, your body is the vehicle that has carried and will continue to carry you through this exciting journey of retirement. Treat it with care, fuel it with good nutrition, and give it the rest it needs. Your body will thank you, and you'll be better equipped to enjoy this beautiful ride called retirement.

4.2 Low-Impact Exercises for Seniors

Maintaining physical activity is a primary ingredient for a healthy retirement, akin to adding a pinch of salt to a favorite recipe. While high-intensity workouts may not be suitable for everyone, low-impact exercises can offer a beneficial alternative, especially for seniors. These types of activities are easy on your joints, can be adapted to your fitness level, and still provide fantastic health benefits. Here, we'll explore three low-impact exercises ideally suited for seniors: walking, swimming, and Tai Chi.

Walking

Consider the simple, rhythmic act of walking. It's as natural as breathing and an activity you've been doing most of your life. Walking is a fantastic low-impact exercise that can be easily integrated into your daily routine. It doesn't require fancy equipment or a gym membership, just a comfortable pair of shoes.

Walking regularly can help strengthen your muscles, improve your balance and coordination, and boost your cardiovascular health. Additionally, it's an excellent way to enjoy the outdoors. You could explore a local park, follow a scenic trail, or even walk around your neighborhood. And when the weather is too hot or raining, you can enjoy a stroll through the mall. A number of the outlet malls have early bird hours for mall walking before the stores open.

If you're just starting, begin with short, manageable distances. Gradually increase your walking time until you reach at least 30 minutes a day. Remember, the goal is not speed but consistency. You could also invite a friend or join a walking group to make the activity more enjoyable.

Swimming

Imagine the gentle lapping of water against the pool edge, the coolness against your skin, and the buoyant feeling as you glide through the water. Swimming is a wonderful, whole-body workout that is easy on your joints.

The buoyancy of the water supports your weight, reducing the strain on your joints and decreasing the risk of injury. It's a great way to increase your heart rate and improve cardiovascular health. Plus, the resistance of the water helps strengthen your muscles without putting too much stress on your body. Our local community center has different classes, from walking laps to swimming laps, water workouts, and water aerobics.

Most local community centers and YMCAs offer swimming classes specifically designed for seniors, providing a safe environment to learn and practice. Whether you're a seasoned swimmer or a beginner, swimming can be an enjoyable and beneficial addition to your exercise routine.

Tai Chi

Imagine standing in a quiet room, your body moving fluidly from one pose to another, your breathing synchronized with your movements. This is Tai Chi, an ancient Chinese martial art often referred to as "meditation in motion."

Tai Chi combines slow, deliberate movements, meditation, and deep breathing. While your body is moving, your mind needs to focus and follow the flow, which can help reduce stress and improve mental clarity.

Tai Chi is particularly beneficial for improving balance and flexibility, two crucial aspects of physical health that can be impacted as we age. The movements are low impact and put minimal stress on muscles and joints, making it safe and effective for seniors.

Local community centers, senior centers, and YMCAs often offer Tai Chi classes for beginners. Learning from a qualified instructor can ensure that you're performing the movements correctly and safely.

Incorporating these low-impact exercises into your routine can greatly enhance your physical well-being. They offer a balanced mix of cardiovascular training, strength building, flexibility, and balance improvement. So, put on your walking shoes, dip your toes in the pool, or find a Tai Chi class near you. It's time to move, to stretch, and to embrace the benefits of staying active in your golden years. Life is meant to be lived actively, regardless of the number of candles on your birthday cake!

4.3 Nutrition for the Golden Years

Consider the act of preparing a delicious, home-cooked meal. You select high-quality ingredients, carefully measure them out, and combine them in just the right way to create a dish that's not only flavorful but also nutritious. Feeding your body, especially as you journey into your golden years, should be no different. Choosing the right 'ingredients' in the form of hydration, fiber-rich foods, and lean proteins can significantly contribute to your health and vitality during retirement.

Hydration

Think about a lush, vibrant plant thriving in your garden, its leaves reaching out towards the sun, its roots firmly anchored into the soil. Now, what's the one thing this plant needs every day to survive and thrive? Water. Much like this plant, our bodies also need water to function properly.

Water plays a vital role in nearly every bodily function. It's crucial for maintaining body temperature, keeping joints lubricated, delivering nutrients to cells, and flushing out waste from the body. As we age, our sense of thirst may decrease, and we might not drink enough fluids, which can lead to dehydration.

Ensuring proper hydration is as simple as having a glass of water within reach throughout the day. Flavoring your water with a slice of lemon or cucumber or drinking herbal teas can also add variety and make hydration more enjoyable. Foods with high water content, such as cucumbers, watermelon, and oranges, can also contribute to your daily water intake.

Fiber-rich foods

Consider a busy highway during rush hour, cars moving at a snail's pace, and traffic backed up for miles. Now picture a clear, open road where vehicles are cruising along smoothly. Dietary fiber can help your digestive system function like that open road, keeping everything moving along smoothly and preventing any 'traffic jams' in your digestive tract.

Fiber, found in foods like fruits, vegetables, whole grains, and legumes, is a crucial part of a healthy diet. It aids in maintaining a healthy weight, managing blood sugar levels, and lowering the risk of heart disease.

Incorporating fiber-rich foods into your diet is as simple as adding a side salad to your lunch, snacking on fresh fruits, or choosing whole-grain bread for your sandwich. Remember, when increasing fiber in your diet, it's important to do so gradually and to increase your water intake as well to avoid any digestive discomfort.

Lean proteins

Consider a team of builders working tirelessly to construct a beautiful house. They need bricks, cement, and other materials to get the job done. In your body, the role of the builder is played by proteins. They are the building blocks of your body, crucial for repairing and building tissues, making hormones and enzymes, and supporting a healthy immune system.

As we age, our bodies need more protein to preserve muscle mass and strength. Lean proteins, like skinless chicken, fish, eggs, beans, and low-fat dairy, can provide this necessary protein without the added saturated fat found in fattier cuts of meat.

Including lean proteins in your diet could be as simple as having a hard-boiled egg for a snack, grilling a piece of salmon for dinner, or adding a handful of black beans to your salad.

Just like that perfect home-cooked meal, a balanced diet in retirement should be a mix of essential 'ingredients' - hydration, fiber-rich foods, and lean proteins. By incorporating these into your meals, you're not only treating your taste buds but also fueling your body with the nutrients it needs to support your active and fulfilling retirement life. So, raise a glass of water, enjoy a fruit salad, and savor a piece of grilled chicken. Your body will thank you, and you'll be better equipped to enjoy this beautiful ride called retirement.

4.4 The Benefits of a Healthy Routine

Think about your favorite song, the one that gets your foot tapping and your heart singing. It has a rhythm, a sequence of beats that creates harmony, a melody. Now, let's apply this melody to our daily lives in the form of a healthy routine. A regular sleep schedule, daily physical activity, and time for relaxation - these are the beats that make up the melody of a healthy lifestyle. Let's take a deeper look into the importance of each 'beat' and how it contributes to our well-being.

Regular Sleep Schedule

Consider the hush that falls over a bustling city at the end of the day, the quiet that blankets the streets as night takes over. This is nature's way of signaling that it's time to rest, to recharge. Maintaining a regular sleep schedule is our way of aligning with this natural rhythm, of giving our bodies the rest they need to function optimally.

A regular sleep schedule means going to bed and waking up at the same time every day, even on weekends. This consistency can regulate your body's internal clock, making it easier to fall asleep and wake up refreshed.

A regular sleep schedule also helps improve the quality of sleep. Good quality sleep can enhance your memory, boost your immune system, and even help manage weight. It's like the night shift crew that comes in to clean, repair, and prepare the city for the next day.

So, make sleep a priority. Create a soothing bedtime routine, make your bedroom a sleep-friendly environment, and stick to a regular sleep schedule. Your body and mind will thank you for it.

Daily Physical Activity

Imagine the gentle sway of trees in the breeze, the fluttering of leaves, the dance of branches. This movement is nature's way of staying flexible, of staying strong. Incorporating physical activity into our daily routine is our way of mirroring this natural movement of keeping our bodies flexible and strong.

Physical activity is not just about maintaining a healthy weight or building muscle strength. It's also about enhancing balance and coordination, boosting mood and energy levels, and promoting better sleep.

Aim for at least 30 minutes of moderate-intensity activity most days of the week. It could be a brisk walk in the park, a swim in the local pool, or a Tai Chi class. Remember, the goal is not intensity but consistency. So, find an activity you enjoy, make it a part of your daily routine, and keep moving.

Time for Relaxation

Have you ever seen a calm, serene lake, its surface smooth and untroubled? It's a picture of tranquility, of peace. Building time for relaxation into our daily routine is our way of creating this tranquility within ourselves, calming our minds and soothing our souls.

Relaxation isn't just about lounging on the couch watching TV. It's about engaging in activities that calm your mind that bring you joy and peace. It could be reading a book, listening to music, meditating, or simply sitting quietly in a garden.

Relaxation helps reduce stress, improve mood, and enhance mental clarity. It's like hitting the reset button on your mental computer, clearing out the clutter, and refreshing the system.

So, make time for relaxation. Dedicate a part of your day to unwind, to do something you enjoy, to simply be. Let this time be your sanctuary, your refuge from the hustle and bustle of life.

A healthy routine is like a well-composed song, with each beat contributing to the overall melody. A regular sleep schedule, daily physical activity, and time for relaxation - these are the beats that make up the rhythm of a healthy retirement life. So, dance to this rhythm, let it guide your days, and experience the harmony it brings to your life.

As we wrap up this chapter, let's take a moment to appreciate the gift of health, the ability to move, to rest, to enjoy life. Let's celebrate this gift by prioritizing our health, creating a routine that promotes well-being, and embracing the habits that keep us fit and healthy. After all, retirement is a time for celebration, for living life to the fullest, and for making every note of this beautiful song count. Stay tuned for the next part of our journey, where we'll explore the social aspects of retirement and how to build and maintain connections in this golden phase of life.

Chapter 5: The Social Aspect: Building and Maintaining Connections

"Stay young at heart, kind in spirit, and enjoy retirement living." –Danielle Duckery

Imagine stepping into a room filled with laughter, lively conversations, and a palpable sense of camaraderie. You see familiar faces and friends who share your interests, understand your jokes, and appreciate your stories. This is your tribe, a group of people who add joy, support, and richness to your life. Now, imagine your retirement life brimming with such interactions, with opportunities to connect, engage, and form meaningful relationships. Sounds wonderful, doesn't it?

In this chapter, we'll explore the value of social engagement in retirement, the joys of joining clubs, the satisfaction of volunteering, and the fun of participating in community events. These are the threads that weave the social fabric of your retirement life, making it colorful, vibrant, and deeply fulfilling.

5.1 The Value of Social Engagement in Retirement

As social beings, we thrive on connections and interactions. They are the lifelines that anchor us, the sparks that ignite joy and a sense of belonging. In retirement, the importance of social engagement gets magnified. Let's understand why.

Joining Clubs

Clubs are like microcosms of the community, offering a platform to meet people, share interests, and indulge in enjoyable activities. Think of a club as a recurring event in your social calendar, something you look forward to and prepare for. The anticipation of the meeting, the discussions, the shared laughter - these not only enhance your mood but also stimulate your mind.

Joining a club can be as simple as reaching out to your local community center or library. Most of them host a variety of clubs catering to different interests. It could be a gardening club, a bird-watching group, or a movie club. The key is to choose a club that aligns with your interests or sparks your curiosity.

Volunteering

Volunteering provides a sense of purpose, a feeling that you're contributing to something bigger than yourself. It's an opportunity to give back to the community to make a difference in the lives of others. The joy of seeing a smile on someone's face, and the satisfaction of knowing you've helped, are feelings that money can't buy.

Volunteering is as versatile as it is rewarding. Love books? Consider volunteering at your local library. Enjoy working with your hands? A community garden could use your help. Passionate about a cause? Numerous non-profit organizations are always looking for volunteers.

Participating in Community Events

Community events are like snapshots of local culture and traditions, offering a glimpse into the spirit of the community. They are platforms for social interaction and places to meet neighbors, make friends, and feel a part of the community.

Participating in community events can be as simple as attending a local concert, a farmer's market, or a holiday parade. These events not only provide entertainment but also create opportunities to connect with people and build relationships.

In essence, social engagement is like the sunshine that brightens our days, the wind that lifts our spirits. It's a vital component of a fulfilling retirement life, one that brings joy, satisfaction, and a sense of belonging. So, take the plunge. Join a club, volunteer for a cause you care about, and participate in community events.

Let your retirement life be filled with meaningful connections, shared laughter, and the warm glow of companionship.

A Picture of Social Engagement

Let's paint a picture of what social engagement could look like in your retirement life. It's a Tuesday morning, and you're at the local community garden, volunteering your time to plant new seedlings. You're surrounded by fellow volunteers, each doing their part to create a green oasis in the heart of the city.

On Wednesday, you're at the local library, attending the monthly meeting of the book club. The book of the month is a gripping mystery novel, and the room is abuzz with theories and discussions. You pitch in with your views, enjoying the animated debate that follows.

Come Friday, and it's time for the annual community fair. You wander through the stalls, enjoy the local cuisine, and even participate in a few fun games. You bump into a couple of your book club members, share a laugh, and promise to catch up at the next meeting.

This is social engagement in retirement - active, engaging, and deeply fulfilling. It's about being a part of a community, about sharing experiences, and about forging bonds that enrich your life. It's about making your golden years truly golden.

5.2 Finding Your Tribe: Clubs and Groups for Seniors

Book Clubs

Imagine a cozy living room, the air filled with the rich aroma of coffee and the rustle of turning pages. Around you, fellow enthusiasts are deep in conversation, dissecting a plot twist, debating a character's motivations, or sharing their favorite passages. This is the magic of book clubs, a gathering that transforms the solitary act of reading into a shared adventure.

Book clubs bring together people who share a love for literature. They offer a platform to explore different genres, discover new authors, and gain fresh perspectives. Each meeting is a journey into a different world, a chance to live a thousand lives through the pages of books.

But the benefits of joining a book club extend beyond the joy of reading. They stimulate intellectual conversations, foster social connections, and often lead to lifelong friendships. In essence, they create a community bound by the love for stories and the joy of sharing them.

So, reach out to your local library or community center to find a book club that suits your literary tastes. Whether you're a fan of classic literature, a lover of mysteries, or a devotee of biographies, there's a book club out there waiting to welcome you.

Gardening Groups

Picture a sunny day, the world bathed in a golden glow, a gentle breeze rustling the leaves. You're kneeling in a garden, your hands deep in the soil, planting seeds that will soon sprout into vibrant flowers or lush vegetables. Around you, fellow gardeners are busy tending their patches, each one a labor of love, a testament to patience and care. This is the beauty of gardening groups, a collective of nature lovers who find joy in the act of growing.

Gardening groups offer a platform to share your love for nature, exchange tips and advice, and learn from fellow gardeners. From discussing the right time to plant tomatoes to identifying that pesky bug eating your roses, each meeting is a treasure trove of knowledge and experiences.

Beyond the joy of gardening, these groups promote physical activity, offer stress relief, and foster a sense of community. They transform gardening from a solitary hobby into a shared passion, a collective effort to bring more green into the world.

So, put on your gardening gloves, pack your trowel and pruning shears, and join a gardening group. Let your love for nature bloom in the company of fellow gardeners.

Art Classes

Imagine a room filled with the scent of paint, the soft scratching of pencils on paper, and the quiet concentration of creativity at work. Around you, fellow artists are engrossed in their creations, each canvas a window into their imagination. This is the allure of art classes, a gathering of creative minds and artistic souls.

Art classes provide an avenue to explore your creativity, learn new techniques, and express yourself through art. Whether you're a seasoned artist or a beginner, these classes offer a supportive environment to nurture your artistic talents.

But art classes are more than just about creating art. They stimulate your imagination, improve your concentration, and provide a sense of accomplishment. They also offer an opportunity to socialize, to share your work, and to gain inspiration from others.

So, pick up your paintbrush, ready your palette, and enroll in an art class. Unleash your creativity, let your canvas tell your story, and let the colors of your art brighten your retirement days.

Remember, finding your tribe and your community in retirement is about more than just filling your calendar. It's about finding shared passions, making connections, and creating a sense of belonging. It's about making your retirement life not just active but also interactive. So, whether it's discussing a book, planting a garden, or painting a canvas, do it in the company of like-minded individuals, in the company of friends. After all, retirement is more fun when shared with others.

Now, let's turn the page and explore another facet of retirement - the joy of giving back, of making a difference, of volunteering. It's a journey into the heart of the community, a journey that's as rewarding as it is fulfilling. So, are you ready to step into this journey, to give back, to touch lives? Let's get started.

5.3 Volunteering: Giving Back to the Community

In the heart of your local town, there's a bustling food bank. Here, volunteers work with a sense of purpose, sorting out donations, filling up grocery bags, and lending a helping hand to those in need. This is one of the several avenues where your retirement years can make a significant difference. When you extend your support to such initiatives, you're not just filling empty stomachs but also filling hearts with hope.

Local Food Banks

Think about a time when a warm meal comforted you, not just with its taste, but with the love with which it was served. Now, imagine sharing that comfort with those who need it the most. Local food banks serve as a crucial lifeline for families and individuals facing food insecurity. They function as a bridge between surplus and need, between abundance and scarcity.

As a volunteer, your role might include sorting and packing food donations, assisting with distribution, or even organizing food drives in your neighborhood. It's an opportunity to play an active role in your community, to witness the direct impact of your efforts, and to meet like-minded individuals committed to the same cause.

Animal Shelters

Picture a playful pup wagging its tail, a purring kitten nuzzling your hand, their eyes filled with trust and affection. Animal shelters are home to countless such creatures, each waiting for a forever home, each with a story to tell. Volunteering at an animal shelter can be an incredibly rewarding experience, one that combines your love for animals with the joy of giving back.

Your role as a volunteer could range from walking dogs and socializing with cats to assisting with adoption events or office tasks. It's a chance to be a part of an animal's journey to a better life, to provide them with care, and to work towards a cause close to your heart.

Community Centers

Envision a vibrant community center buzzing with activities. Children learning to paint, seniors practicing yoga, and teenagers engrossed in a coding workshop. Community centers are like the heartbeat of a neighborhood, offering a plethora of activities for residents of all ages.

Volunteering at a community center can open doors to a multitude of experiences. You could help organize events, teach a class based on your skills, or assist in maintaining the center. It's a way to connect with your neighbors, to contribute to local development, and to create a positive environment for learning and recreation.

In the grand tapestry of retirement, volunteering is a thread that adds depth and richness. It's a path that leads you to the heart of your community, a path marked by kindness, compassion, and a sense of purpose. So, step into a food bank, an animal shelter, or a community center, and let the magic of volunteering color your retirement years with hues of fulfillment and joy.

5.4 Maintaining Connections: Friends and Family

Picture a warm Sunday afternoon, the air filled with the tantalizing aroma of a backyard barbecue, the sound of laughter, and lively chatter echoing around. You're surrounded by your loved ones - your children, grandchildren, siblings, and lifelong friends. This is the essence of retirement - the freedom to spend precious moments with those who matter most, and to nurture connections that span a lifetime.

Regular Visits

Like a beautiful garden that flourishes with regular care and attention, relationships, too, thrive on frequent interactions. Regular visits to your friends and loved ones can keep these connections alive and vibrant. These visits don't have to be elaborate. They could be as simple as a cup of coffee at a neighborhood café, a walk in the park, or a shared meal at home.

These visits offer a platform for heart-to-heart conversations, shared laughter, and the joy of simply being in each other's company. They serve as a reminder of the bonds you share, the memories you've created, and the love that binds you together. So, mark your calendar, plan a visit, and let the warmth of these interactions add a glow to your retirement days.

Family Gatherings

Now, imagine a large dining table, groaning under the weight of delicious dishes, surrounded by your family. There's the clinking of glasses, the swapping of stories, and the comfort of being with family. Family gatherings are like the high notes in the symphony of life, moments that resonate with joy, love, and togetherness.

These gatherings could be for special occasions like birthdays and anniversaries, or they could be 'just because' get-togethers. They're opportunities to create memories, to celebrate milestones, and to strengthen the bonds that tie your family together.

Family gatherings are also a platform for bridging the generation gap, for sharing wisdom and experiences with the younger generation, and for learning about their world. They're a celebration of the family you've built, the legacy you've created. So, plan that family barbecue, host that holiday dinner, and let these gatherings be the highlights of your retirement life.

Virtual Meet-ups

In today's digital age, staying connected is just a click away. Virtual meet-ups offer a convenient and flexible way to maintain connections, especially with loved ones who live far away. All you need is a device with an internet connection, and you can video call your friends and family, no matter where they are in the world.

Virtual meet-ups can be as warm and engaging as in-person interactions. You could have a virtual coffee date with a friend, read bedtime stories to your grandkids, or even watch a movie together using streaming platforms.

Embracing technology for social interactions can open up new avenues for maintaining connections. It's a testament to the fact that distance doesn't define relationships, and love transcends all boundaries. So, set up that video call, dial that number, and let your voice and your smile brighten up your loved ones' day.

In the grand scheme of retirement, maintaining connections is like keeping the home fires burning, providing warmth, light, and a sense of belonging. These connections - with friends, family, and the community - form the heart of your retirement life. They add love, joy, and richness to your golden years. They remind you that no matter where you are in life, it's the people you share it with that make it truly meaningful.

As the sun sets on this chapter, let's take a moment to appreciate the bonds we share with our loved ones, the joy these connections bring, and the love that makes our world go round. These are the treasures that we carry in our hearts, the treasures that make our retirement life truly priceless. So, here's to love, laughter, and a lifetime of connections. Let's step into it with open hearts and minds, ready to embrace the adventures that await us.

Chapter 6 Embrace Life's New Chapter with Travel

"My parents didn't want to move to Florida, but they turned sixty, and that's the law." –Jerry Seinfeld

As the early morning sun peeks through your window, you find yourself not reaching for the alarm clock but for the suitcase at the end of your bed. The smell of adventure is in the air. Retirement has opened up a new world of travel possibilities. The door to the unknown stands ajar, waiting for you to step through. There's a whole planet out there to explore, cultures to immerse yourself in, and experiences waiting to be had. Let's start with understanding why traveling during retirement can be such a rewarding endeavor.

6.1 Benefits of Traveling in Retirement

Broadened Horizons

Stepping into a foreign land, hearing the lilt of a new language, tasting unfamiliar cuisine, and witnessing age-old traditions can be an enlightening experience. Travel has a way of broadening your horizons, of making you see the world in a new light. It breaks down barriers, shatters stereotypes, and fosters a sense of global unity. Think of it like reading a book, but instead of turning pages, you're traversing the globe, absorbing life lessons along the way.

Enhanced Mental Stimulation

Navigating through unfamiliar streets, learning a few phrases in a new language, or understanding a different culture – travel is a mental workout. It challenges your adaptability, problem-solving skills, and cognitive flexibility. It's like a puzzle, where you're piecing together different elements to create a memorable experience. This mental stimulation can keep your brain active and sharp, which is crucial in maintaining cognitive health during retirement.

Improved Physical Health

Whether it's hiking through a national park, strolling through a city's historic district, or swimming in the clear waters of a tropical beach, travel often involves a degree of physical activity. This can boost your cardiovascular health, improve flexibility, and even strengthen your immune system. Picture yourself exploring the winding paths of a beautiful garden in Paris or walking along the Great Wall of China. These activities not only satisfy your wanderlust but also contribute to your fitness goals.

Strengthened Relationships

Traveling with a partner, family, or friends can strengthen bonds. Shared experiences, whether it's marveling at a beautiful sunset or navigating through a bustling foreign market, create lasting memories. These shared moments can bring you closer, fostering understanding and deepening emotional connections. Imagine a family trip where your grandchildren learn about their heritage or a getaway with friends where old memories are revisited and new ones are created.

Increased Happiness and Satisfaction

There's a certain joy in planning a trip, the anticipation of what's to come. Then there's the pleasure of the trip itself, the daily discoveries, and experiences. And finally, there's the joy of reminiscing, of looking back at the photos and reliving the memories. Each stage of travel increases happiness and life satisfaction. It gives you something to look forward to, something to experience, and something to look back on. It's a cycle of joy, keeping your spirits high and your heart full.

So, dust off your suitcase, pack your curiosity and sense of adventure, and get ready to explore the world. Remember, the world is a book, and those who do not travel read only one page. It's time to turn the page and start a new chapter in your retirement life, a chapter filled with adventures, discoveries, and priceless experiences.

6.2 Planning Your Travel: Tips and Tricks

Researching Destinations

Unfolding a world map, letting your finger glide over continents and oceans, your mind buzzing with possibilities - selecting your travel destination is the first exciting step in your adventure. But the choice can be overwhelming. A little research can make this process easier, more enjoyable, and ultimately more rewarding.

Start by asking yourself what you seek from your travels. Are you yearning for sun-kissed beaches or snow-capped mountains? Do you wish to immerse yourself in rich history and culture, or would you prefer a place buzzing with modernity and innovation?

Once you've narrowed down your preferences, dig deeper into the specifics of each potential destination. Look up the best time to visit, local customs and traditions, available amenities, and the must-see spots. Don't forget to check out traveler reviews and forums for firsthand insights.

Budgeting for Travel

While the idea of a no-expense-spared vacation might seem appealing, a well-planned budget ensures that your travel plans don't strain your retirement fund. A travel budget is not just about controlling expenses; it's about optimizing your travel experience without financial stress.

Start by listing down all possible expenses - flights, accommodation, meals, sightseeing, shopping, and even gratuities. Next, allocate an estimated amount to each expense. Be realistic and always factor in some contingency funds for unexpected costs.

Remember, a budget is a tool for planning, not a rigid financial constraint. It should serve as a guide, helping you make informed decisions and prioritize your spending.

Booking in Advance

Securing your travel arrangements well in advance can save you both money and stress. Early bird flight tickets and hotel bookings often come at discounted rates. Moreover, advance booking ensures availability, especially during peak tourist seasons.

While booking, compare prices on different websites and consider package deals that bundle flights, hotels, and even sightseeing tours. Don't forget to read the fine print, particularly the cancellation and refund policies.

Remember, the goal of advance booking is not just to snag a deal; it's about ensuring a smooth and hassle-free travel experience.

Packing Essentials

Imagine opening your suitcase upon arrival to find everything you need neatly packed and easily accessible. Efficient packing can make your travel experience more comfortable and convenient.

Start by making a list of essentials - clothing suitable for the weather, toiletries, medications, travel documents, and any other items you use daily. It's beneficial to pack versatile clothing items that you can mix and match.

Invest in travel-sized toiletries or reusable travel bottles to save space. Most importantly, ensure all essential documents, including passport, ID, travel insurance, and emergency contact details, are stored safely and are easily accessible.

A well-packed suitcase is like your personal travel kit, equipped to make your journey comfortable and carefree.

Travel Insurance Considerations

Travel insurance is like a safety net, offering protection against unforeseen circumstances during your travels. It typically covers medical emergencies, trip cancellations, lost luggage, and other unexpected travel-related costs.

Before purchasing travel insurance, evaluate your needs and the level of risk. Consider factors like the length and nature of your trip, your health condition, and the coverage of any existing insurance policies.

Choose a policy that offers comprehensive coverage tailored to your needs. Ensure to understand the terms and conditions, including the claim process and what's not covered.

Retirement is your ticket to explore the world at your own pace, to immerse in new experiences, and to create a suitcase full of memories. As you gear up for this exciting phase, remember that successful travel requires more than just a destination; it requires careful planning and preparation. So, put on your planner's hat, take the first step, and let the thrill of travel fill your retirement days with adventure, discovery, and joy.

6.3 Travel Ideas for Every Budget

Retirement is a golden ticket to a world waiting to be discovered, and the best part is it doesn't have to break the bank. There are travel options to suit every budget, each with its unique charm and experiences. Let's explore some of these options, shall we?

Road Trips

There's something special about hitting the open road with the wind in your hair and a map in your glove compartment. Road trips offer a sense of freedom and adventure that's hard to match. You set the pace, choose the stops, and soak in the changing landscapes as you cruise along.

Road trips can be surprisingly budget-friendly. You save on airfare, and with a little planning, you can find affordable accommodation or even camp under the stars. Pack a picnic basket, and you've got your meals covered too. The journey is as important as the destination on a road trip. So whether it's a scenic coastal drive or an epic cross-country adventure, road trips are perfect for the budget-conscious traveler.

Voluntourism

Imagine helping to build a school in a remote village or volunteering at a wildlife conservation project. This is what voluntourism is all about – combining travel with volunteering. It's a chance to give back to the community while exploring new places.

Voluntourism often includes accommodation and meals, which can make it a cost-effective way to travel. Plus, it provides a unique perspective of the destination, far removed from the regular tourist trail. It's an experience that enriches not just your travel album but also your soul.

Staycations

Who says you need to travel far to have a great vacation? Sometimes, the best adventures can be found right in your backyard. A staycation is all about exploring your local area as a tourist. Visit museums, enjoy parks, try out new restaurants, or even book a couple of nights in a local hotel for a change of scenery.

Staycations can be a real budget-saver. You save on travel costs and yet get to enjoy the perks of being on vacation. Plus, it's a fantastic way to discover and appreciate the gems in your local area.

Group Tours

Traveling solo can be an amazing experience, but group tours offer their own set of advantages. They take the hassle out of planning, provide company, and often work out cheaper as costs are shared.

Group tours often include accommodation, transportation, and most meals, making it easier to budget for your trip. They also provide a sense of safety, which can be a big plus if you're traveling to a new destination. Whether it's a historical tour of

Europe or a wildlife safari in Africa, group tours offer a social and cost-effective way to travel.

Cruises

Imagine waking up to a different view from your window each morning – one day, it's a bustling port city; the next, it's a peaceful island beach. Cruises offer an all-inclusive vacation on the sea, with meals, entertainment, and accommodation all on one ship.

While cruises can seem pricey at first glance, they offer great value for money, considering what's included. Plus, there are options for every budget, from luxury liners to budget-friendly cruises. So, set sail on the high seas for a vacation that combines relaxation, exploration, and great value.

Whether you're cruising the highways on a road trip, volunteering in a distant land, playing tourist in your hometown, joining a group tour, or sailing the high seas, retirement is your chance to quench your wanderlust without draining your wallet. It's a time to collect experiences, not things. To make memories that will warm your heart in the years to come. Here's to affordable adventures and priceless experiences in your retirement years.

6.4 Travel Safety Tips for Seniors

Regular Health Checks

Imagine you're getting ready to take your dream car for a long drive. You'd first ensure it's in top condition, right? You'd check the tires, the engine, the brakes, and the oil. Similarly, before embarking on your travel adventures, you need to ensure your health is in optimal condition, too.

Regular health checks are crucial in this regard. Before any trip, schedule an appointment with your doctor for a general check-up. Discuss your travel plans, the destinations you'll be visiting, and any potential health risks associated with them. This is also a good time to discuss any vaccinations you might need for specific destinations.

Medication Management

On any journey, a well-stocked first aid kit is a must-have. But for seniors, it's also important to manage regular medications. Start by making a list of the medications you take, along with their dosages. Keep this list with you at all times during your travel.

If you take prescription medications, make sure you have enough to last the duration of the trip, plus a little extra in case of travel delays. Keep medications in their original packaging to avoid confusion, and carry a copy of the prescription as well.

Remember to adjust your medication schedule according to any change in time zones and set reminders so you don't miss a dose. A well-planned medication regimen can help maintain your health and well-being while you're exploring the world.

Emergency Contacts

An explorer always has a compass, a reliable tool that points the way in case they lose their path. For a senior traveler, an emergency contact list is that vital compass. It should include the phone numbers of family members, your doctor, and your health insurance provider.

Also, research the emergency services contact numbers for your destination, such as the local ambulance, fire department, and the nearest embassy or consulate if you're traveling internationally.

Keep this list both in a digital format on your phone and as a physical copy in your wallet. This ensures you have access to these crucial numbers even if your phone battery dies or you lose your phone.

Travel Scam Awareness

Just as a seasoned sailor is aware of potential storms and navigates to avoid them, a smart traveler must be aware of common travel scams. These scams could range from overpriced taxi rides and 'free' gifts to more serious ones like identity theft.

Before your trip, research common scams at your destination. Always keep your personal belongings secure, be wary of unsolicited offers for assistance, and avoid sharing personal information with strangers.

Stay vigilant, trust your instincts, and don't let anyone rush you into making a decision. An informed and alert traveler is less likely to fall victim to scams, ensuring your travel experience remains positive and stress-free.

Safe and savvy traveling is like creating a beautiful piece of art. It involves careful preparation, constant awareness, and a touch of creativity. By managing your health, organizing your medications, preparing an emergency contact list, and staying vigilant about potential scams, you can ensure that your travel experiences are not just enjoyable but also safe and secure. So, fasten your seatbelt, rev up your engine, and let the road of travel unfold before you. Just around the corner, new experiences, discoveries, and adventures await you.

Chapter 7: Igniting Your Creativity: Arts, Crafts, and More

"Retirement gives you the time literally to recreate yourself through a sport, game or hobby that you always wanted to try or that you haven't done in years." –Steven Price

Imagine the feeling of a paintbrush gliding smoothly across a canvas, each stroke adding color, life, and meaning to a once-blank space. Or the rhythm of knitting needles clicking together, weaving yarn into a warm, cozy blanket. Picture the joy of strumming a guitar, each note resonating with your mood, echoing in your soul. These moments of creative expression are magical, aren't they? They are moments when time seems to stand still, when the mind is focused, and the heart is content.

Creativity is not just for artists or musicians. It's a part of everyone's life, a source of joy, fulfillment, and personal growth. As we step into the golden years of retirement, we have the freedom to explore this creativity, to immerse ourselves in the arts, crafts, music, and dance, and to express ourselves in ways we never thought possible. So, let's dive into this colorful world of creativity and discover the boundless joy it can bring into our retirement life.

7.1 The Joy of Creative Expression

Stress Relief

Creating art, whether it's painting a landscape, crafting a piece of jewelry, or playing a musical instrument, can be an incredibly calming experience. It's like taking a break from the hustle and bustle of everyday life, stepping into a peaceful sanctuary where the mind can relax and the spirit can rejuvenate. The act of focusing on an art project can help reduce stress, much like meditation. So, the next time you're feeling stressed, why not pick up a paintbrush or a piece of clay and let your creativity flow?

Cognitive Function Boost

Engaging in creative activities can also give your brain a good workout. When you learn a new craft technique, master a tricky piano piece, or design a piece of jewelry, you're challenging your brain, enhancing your problem-solving skills, and improving your cognitive function. Think of it as a fun and enjoyable brain exercise that not only stimulates your grey cells but also results in a beautiful piece of art or music.

Emotional Outlet

Artistic expression can also serve as an emotional outlet, a way to express feelings that are hard to put into words. A splash of red paint might represent your passion, a melancholy tune on the piano might echo your sadness, and a piece of handmade jewelry might symbolize your love for a dear one. By expressing these emotions through art, you're not only creating something beautiful but also processing your feelings in a healthy and therapeutic way.

Sense of Accomplishment

There's a unique sense of accomplishment in creating something with your own hands, isn't there? The pride of seeing your painting displayed on the wall, the joy of wearing a sweater you've knitted, the satisfaction of playing a song on the guitar - these are rewards that money can't buy. They boost your self-esteem, enhance your self-confidence, and give you a sense of achievement.

Social Connection

Last but definitely not least, engaging in creative activities can be a great way to socialize. Joining a painting class, a craft group, or a choir can provide opportunities to meet like-minded people, share ideas, and form new friendships. These social interactions add a whole new dimension to your creative pursuits, making them even more enjoyable and fulfilling.

In conclusion, creative expression in retirement is like adding a splash of color to a canvas, a melody to a silent room, and a spark of joy to everyday life. It's a path to stress relief, cognitive stimulation, emotional expression, personal accomplishment, and social connection. So, go ahead, explore your creativity, let your imagination soar, and let your retirement life be a beautiful masterpiece of your own making. Just remember, in this creative journey, there are no mistakes, only unique creations. Now, let's delve deeper into the world of art and discover how it can enrich our retirement lives.

7.2 Discovering Art: Painting, Sculpture, and More

Watercolor Painting

Imagine a blank canvas waiting to be transformed into a riot of colors and emotions. Watercolor painting is all about letting your imagination take flight. With a palette of vibrant hues and a brush as your wand, you can create landscapes, portraits, or abstract pieces that reflect your inner world.

Getting started with watercolor painting is quite simple. All you need are some basic supplies – watercolor paints, brushes, and watercolor paper. Start by playing around with the colors, understanding how they blend and how water impacts their intensity. As you gain confidence, you can start working on simple projects and gradually move on to more complex compositions. Remember, every stroke, every splash of color, is a step forward in your artistic exploration.

Pottery Making

Feel the cool, pliable clay beneath your fingers, watch as it transforms from a shapeless lump into a beautiful pot under the guidance of your hands. Pottery making is not just about creating ceramic pieces; it's a therapeutic process that calms the mind and soothes the soul.

Pottery classes for beginners are a great place to start. They provide hands-on experience, guidance from skilled instructors, and the chance to learn various techniques, from hand-building to wheel throwing. As you shape the clay, you're not just creating a piece of art; you're also shaping a new skill, a new passion.

Collage Art

A snip here, a cut there, and a whole lot of gluing - creating a collage is like piecing together a puzzle. Each piece, be it a photograph, a newspaper clipping, or a piece of fabric, holds a special place in the artwork. The beauty of collage art lies in its simplicity and the endless possibilities it offers.

To start a collage, all you need is a base (like a canvas or a piece of cardboard), some cutouts from magazines or newspapers, photographs, ribbons, or anything else you wish to include in your artwork, and glue. Arrange the pieces on your base, play around with their placement until you're satisfied, and then glue them down. The result is a unique piece of art that tells a story – your story.

Charcoal Drawing

Imagine a piece of charcoal gracefully dancing across a paper, leaving behind a trail of black, creating shapes, shadows, and textures. Charcoal drawing is a versatile and accessible art form. It's about playing with light and shadow, creating depth, and bringing your subject to life.

Charcoal comes in various forms - pencils for detailed work, sticks for bold and broad strokes, and powder for large areas and gradients. Start with basic shapes and gradually move on to complex subjects. The key is to be patient with yourself and enjoy the process of learning and creating.

Origami

A single sheet of paper, folded meticulously, transforming into a beautiful crane, a blooming flower, or a soaring airplane - that's the magic of Origami. This traditional Japanese art form is all about precision, patience, and creativity.

Origami can be as simple or as complex as you want it to be. Start with basic folds and simple models, and as you get the hang of it, you can try more intricate designs. The process of folding paper can be meditative, and the satisfaction of seeing a flat sheet of paper transform into a 3D model is immeasurable.

Art brings color to our lives, adds a dash of creativity to our daily routine, and offers a unique way to express ourselves. It's a testament to the human spirit, our ability to create beauty, to tell stories, and to connect with our inner selves. Retirement offers the perfect canvas to explore this creativity, experiment with different art forms, and discover the artist within. So, pick up that paintbrush, mold that clay, create that collage, draw with charcoal, and fold that paper. Let your creativity shine, let your art tell your story, and let your retirement life be a masterpiece of your own making.

7.3 Crafting Your Way to Happiness

Imagine sitting in a comfortable armchair, a soft ball of yarn in your lap and a pair of knitting needles in your hands. As you weave the yarn into intricate patterns, your mind unwinds, letting go of stress and finding peace in the rhythmic motion. This is the beauty of crafts – a harmonious blend of creativity, relaxation, and pleasure. In this section, let's explore various crafting activities that can add a dash of color, a touch of creativity, and a whole lot of happiness to your retirement life.

Knitting and Crocheting

Knitting and crocheting are like crafting wonders with yarn. With a pair of needles or a hook, you can transform a simple yarn into cozy scarves, cute baby booties, or even plush toys. The process is soothing, almost meditative, and the end result is a handmade item brimming with warmth and love.

Starting with knitting or crocheting is quite simple. All you need is some yarn, knitting needles, a crochet hook, and a beginner's pattern. As your skills improve, you can experiment with different patterns, stitches, and yarn types. Whether you're knitting a sweater for your grandchild or crocheting a blanket for a friend, the joy of creating something with your own hands is incomparable.

And just in case you are wondering, men do crochet and knit too. There is a huge following of men who have been making a name for themselves with crocheting and knitting. Several began learning as they watched their mom or grandmother, others learned by watching YouTube videos during COVID lockdown;

however, some learned out of necessity because they wanted warm scarfs or beanies for winter. They are referred to as sew bros.

Jewelry Making

Consider the sparkle of a bead, the sheen of a metal charm, and the delicate thread that holds them together. Jewelry making is an art that combines creativity, precision, and a keen eye for detail. From elegant necklaces and trendy bracelets to statement earrings and unique brooches, the possibilities are endless.

Starting a jewelry-making hobby requires some basic tools and materials, like beads, charms, wires, and pliers. As you explore this craft, you'll learn various techniques, like wire wrapping, beading, and macramé. The best part? You'll have a collection of custom-made jewelry to wear or gift to your loved ones.

Scrapbooking

Scrapbooking is like weaving stories with photographs, embellishments, and handwritten notes. It's a creative way to preserve memories, document life events, and express your personal style. A scrapbook page can be a vibrant collage of a family vacation, a tender homage to a loved one, or a nostalgic journey into the past.

Starting a scrapbook project is as simple as gathering some photographs, buying a scrapbook album, and letting your creativity guide you. You can add embellishments like stickers, ribbons, and stamps or use patterned paper to make your pages pop. Each page you create is a testament to your life's story, a keepsake for generations to cherish.

Quilting

Quilting is the art of sewing together different pieces of fabric to create a larger design. It's like putting together a jigsaw puzzle, where each piece contributes to the larger picture. A quilt can be a cozy blanket, a vibrant wall hanging, or a cherished heirloom.

Starting a quilting project requires some basic sewing skills, a sewing machine, fabric, batting, and thread. There are various quilting techniques, from traditional patchwork and appliqué to modern art quilting. Whether you're making a baby quilt for your grandchild or a wall hanging for your home, quilting offers a fulfilling and creative outlet.

DIY Home Decor

Imagine transforming a plain vase into a stunning centerpiece or turning reclaimed wood into a rustic shelf. DIY home decor is about seeing the potential in everyday objects and using your creativity to transform them. It's about adding a personal touch to your home, making it a reflection of your style and personality.

DIY home decor projects can range from painting furniture and creating wall art to sewing cushion covers and making wreaths. All you need is an idea, some materials, and a willingness to try. And the result? A home that's filled with unique decor items, each telling its own story, each a testament to your creativity.

In the palette of retirement life, crafting activities add vibrant colors, unique textures, and a whole lot of creativity. They offer a way to relax, to express yourself, and to create beautiful items that bring joy to you and your loved ones. So, pick up those knitting needles, string those beads, gather your photographs, thread that needle, and roll up your sleeves. Let your creativity shine, let your crafts tell your story, and let your retirement life be a beautiful mosaic of experiences, memories, and handmade treasures.

7.4 Music and Dance: A Celebration of Life

Learning a Musical Instrument

Picture yourself seated comfortably, a guitar cradled in your arms. As your fingers glide over the strings, a melody comes to life, filling the air with music. Learning a musical instrument in retirement can be a rewarding experience. It allows you to engage your mind, stimulate your senses, and create something beautiful. Whether it's a piano, a violin, or a ukulele, the instrument you choose becomes a medium for self-expression, an extension of your emotions.

Taking up a musical instrument can be as simple as enrolling in a local music class or seeking online tutorials. The key is to start with the basics and gradually improve your skills. With practice, you'll not only learn to play your favorite tunes but also experience the sheer joy of creating music.

Joining a Choir

Imagine standing amidst a group of people, their voices rising and falling in perfect harmony, creating a symphony of sounds. Joining a choir can be a soulful journey into the world of music. It's an opportunity to lend your voice to a collective melody, to be a part of something that transcends individual notes.

Being a part of a choir is not just about singing; it's also about listening, blending your voice with others, and creating a harmonious sound. It's a chance to socialize, to share the love for music, and to create beautiful memories. Local community centers, churches, and even online platforms offer various choir groups that cater to different musical styles and proficiency levels.

Ballroom Dancing

Visualize a grand ballroom, the air charged with excitement, music filling the corners, and couples swaying to the rhythm. Ballroom dancing is about elegance, coordination, and a whole lot of fun. It's a dance form that's as much about the connection with your partner as it is about the steps.

Joining a ballroom dance class can be a great way to stay active, improve balance, and meet new people. From the lively steps of the Jive to the smooth movements of the Waltz, each dance style offers a unique experience. Plus, it's an excellent opportunity to dress up and enjoy the glamour and sophistication associated with this dance form.

Line Dancing

Think of a room full of people, all moving in unison, following a sequence of steps to the beat of the music. That's the beauty of line dancing. It's a dance form that's fun and social and doesn't require a partner.

Line dancing classes are a great way to keep fit, learn new dance moves, and enjoy a variety of music styles. The steps are easy to follow, making it suitable for individuals of all ages and fitness levels. So, put on your dancing shoes, get in line, and dance your way to happiness.

Music Appreciation Clubs

Envision a comfortable living room, a group of music lovers gathered around, listening to a symphony, discussing its nuances, and appreciating its beauty. Music appreciation clubs offer a platform for music enthusiasts to share their love for music, explore different genres, and deepen their understanding of music.

These clubs organize a range of activities, from listening sessions and discussions to attending concerts or meeting musicians. Being a part of these clubs can enhance your music listening experience, broaden your musical horizons, and provide an opportunity to connect with fellow music lovers.

Life in retirement is like a beautiful song, a melody composed of various notes. Learning a musical instrument, joining a choir, dancing, and appreciating music are like notes that add rhythm, harmony, and joy to your retirement life. So, strum that guitar, hit those high notes, dance like no one's watching, and let the music play. Let your retirement life be a celebration of life, a symphony of memorable experiences, and a dance of joy and contentment.

A Final Note

As we wrap up this chapter, let's embrace the creative spirit within us. Let's dance to the rhythm of our hearts, paint with the colors of our souls, and create crafts that tell our unique story. After all, retirement is a journey of self-discovery, a time to explore new interests, and an opportunity to express our creativity. So, let's pick up the brush, the yarn, the guitar, or the dancing shoes, and let's immerse ourselves in the joy of creative expression. It's time to add our unique touch to the canvas of life.

Chapter 8: Navigating the Cyberspace: Embrace the Digital Age

"While retirement offers the promise of leisure and relaxation, let's not forget the importance of safeguarding our digital lives. In this age of technology, securing our online presence is as vital as ever, ensuring that we enjoy the digital world safely and securely during our retirement years."

We live in an era where the world is at our fingertips, literally. With a few taps on a keyboard or screen, we can connect with friends across the globe, learn a new language, or even take a virtual tour of a museum. Yes, the digital world can seem overwhelming, especially if you're not quite tech-savvy. Whether you retired from a job that had you using technology every day or you are new to it altogether, the truth is updates, changes, and patches are issued every day to make improvements or deal with security issues. Let's not forget that every master was once a beginner. Becoming comfortable with technology starts with taking that first step, and that's what we'll explore in this chapter. Let's get started, shall we?

8.1 Overcoming the Tech Fear: It's Easier Than You Think

Technology is merely a tool, not a mystical entity to be feared. Think of it like mastering the art of driving. Initially, it seems daunting, with so many things to remember and manage simultaneously. But with practice, it becomes second nature. Similarly, overcoming the fear of technology is all about practice and patience. Here are some ways to get started.

Tech Literacy Classes

Remember the excitement of attending your first dance class or the curiosity when you enrolled in that pottery workshop? Why not bring that same enthusiasm to learning technology? Tech literacy classes are designed to help beginners understand and use technology effectively.

These classes cover the basics, from using a computer or smartphone to email basics to navigating the internet. Check your local community centers or libraries for these classes. Some organizations even offer free classes specifically designed for seniors.

One-on-One Tech Tutoring

Learning in a group can be fun, but sometimes, you need that extra attention to grasp a concept. That's where one-on-one tech tutoring can be beneficial. Just like a personal trainer at the gym customizes your workout routine, a tech tutor tailors the lessons to suit your needs and pace.

The beauty of one-on-one tutoring is that you can ask as many questions as you want without feeling self-conscious. You can focus on specific areas you find challenging and learn at your own pace. Look for services in your local community or consider online platforms that offer personalized tech tutoring.

Online Tech Resources

The internet is a treasure trove of information. There are countless websites, video tutorials, and online forums dedicated to helping people become more tech-savvy. Websites like TechBoomers, SeniorNet, and AARP have sections dedicated to technology learning. They offer free tutorials on everything from using social media and online banking to operating your smartphone.

YouTube is another fantastic platform where you can find tutorials on virtually any tech-related topic. The advantage of these resources is that you can pause, rewind, and rewatch these tutorials as many times as you want, learning at your own pace.

Tech Help Hotlines

Remember those times when you needed some advice, and you picked up the phone and called a friend? Tech help hotlines are like that friend, ready to help whenever you're stuck. Most tech companies have a dedicated customer service line to assist with any issues you might face.

Whether you can't log into your email account, your computer is acting up, or an error message pops up that you don't understand, these tech hotlines can help. Keep a list of these numbers handy so you know who to call when you need tech help.

In conclusion, overcoming the fear of technology is not about becoming an expert overnight. It's about taking small steps, practicing regularly, and having the patience to keep learning. It's about making technology your friend, a tool that adds convenience, connection, and learning opportunities to your life. Remember, every online journey begins with a single click. So take that click, embrace the digital age, and let the world of technology enrich your retirement years.

8.2 Learning Online: Platforms and Opportunities

Online Courses

The digital world offers an array of learning opportunities right at your fingertips. Online courses cover a wide range of subjects, from history and philosophy to photography and cooking. Websites like Coursera, Khan Academy, and Udemy host thousands of courses taught by experts in their fields. You can find beginner-friendly courses, intermediate-level, or even advanced courses, depending on your current knowledge and interest.

The beauty of online courses lies in their flexibility. You can learn at your own pace, at a time that suits you, from the comfort of your home. Most courses offer video lectures, reading materials, and quizzes to ensure a comprehensive learning experience. Some even provide certificates upon completion, which can be a great addition to your achievements during retirement.

Virtual Book Clubs

For those who love to read, virtual book clubs can be a fantastic way to share your thoughts and engage in stimulating discussions. Websites like Goodreads and Bookclubz offer platforms where you can join existing book clubs or start your own.

These online clubs choose a book every month, giving members ample time to read. Then, through forum discussions or live video chats, members share their views, discuss themes and characters, and gain diverse perspectives. It's like a gathering of friends, but instead of a café, you meet in cyberspace.

Webinars and Podcasts

Webinars and podcasts have emerged as popular mediums for learning and entertainment. Webinars are live or recorded online seminars on a specific topic. Websites like Eventbrite list a variety of webinars you can join, some free and some paid.

Podcasts, on the other hand, are like radio shows that you can download and listen to on demand. Platforms like Spotify and Apple Podcasts host podcasts on a myriad of topics. Whether you're interested in history, science, travel, or even comedy, there's a podcast out there that caters to your interests.

Virtual Museum Tours

If you appreciate art and history, virtual museum tours can be your passport to the world's most renowned museums. Institutions like The Louvre, The British Museum, and The Metropolitan Museum of Art offer virtual tours of their exhibits.

These tours allow you to explore the museum at your leisure, with detailed descriptions and sometimes even audio guides. It's like having a private viewing of the world's greatest treasures, all from the comfort of your home.

In the realm of the digital world, learning has no boundaries. It offers avenues to explore new subjects, indulge your interests, and even meet like-minded individuals. The plethora of online platforms and opportunities ensures that your retirement years can be as enlightening as they are enjoyable. So, sign up for that online course, join that virtual book club, tune in to that podcast, and embark on a virtual tour of a museum. The world of knowledge is waiting for you.

8.3 Staying Connected: Social Media for Seniors

Picture yourself sipping a cup of coffee, a tablet in your hand, scrolling through a screen filled with updates from friends, interesting articles, and stunning photographs. This is the world of social media, a virtual platform that keeps you connected with loved ones, informed about the world, and engaged with your interests. Let's explore the various social media platforms and how they can enhance your digital experience in retirement.

Facebook Groups for Seniors

Imagine a virtual gathering of people your age, all sharing their retirement experiences, offering advice, and providing support. Facebook groups serve as online communities where people with similar interests can connect and interact. These groups can range from hobby-focused groups and travel clubs for seniors to general discussion groups where you can chat about life, retirement, and everything in between.

Joining a Facebook group is like adding a social event to your digital calendar. It's a space where you can share your thoughts, participate in discussions, and even make new friends. It's a reminder that no matter where you are, you're not alone in your retirement journey.

Video Calling with Skype or Zoom

Think back to a time when hearing the voice of a distant loved one required waiting for a letter or a long-distance call. Today, technology allows us to see and hear our loved ones in real time, no matter how far they are. Video calling platforms like Skype and Zoom have made this possible.

Whether it's a quick chat with your friend who lives across town or a family reunion with relatives scattered across the globe, video calls can make you feel like you're in the same room. It's more personal than a phone call, and the joy of seeing your loved ones' faces is unmatched.

Sharing Photos on Instagram

Envision a digital photo album where you can share your travel snapshots, pictures of your latest knitting project, or even your everyday moments. Instagram offers just that. It's a platform where you can share photos, connect with family and friends, and even follow accounts that interest you, like gardening tips, recipe pages, or inspirational quotes.

The best part of Instagram is the ease of use. Just snap a photo, add a filter if you like, write a caption, and hit share. It's a fun and interactive way to share your retirement adventures and peek into the lives of your loved ones.

Following News on X (formerly Twitter)

Keeping up with current events and news is like maintaining a pulse on the world's heartbeat. Twitter makes this easy. It's a platform where news outlets, journalists, and even world leaders share updates in real time.

Following news on X is like having a personalized newspaper where you can choose what kind of news you want to see, comment on updates, and even share your thoughts. It's a quick and convenient way to stay informed and engaged with world events.

In the vibrant landscape of the digital world, social media platforms are like bustling town squares. They offer spaces to connect, share, and engage with a global community. Navigating these platforms can be a fun and fulfilling part of your retirement routine. So, join that Facebook group, make that video call, share that photo, and tweet your thoughts. The world of social media is waiting to welcome you with open arms and a wealth of connections.

8.4 Digital Safety: Protecting Yourself Online

As exciting as the digital world is, it's equally important to navigate it safely. Just as you lock your doors at night or buckle your seatbelt before driving, certain precautions ensure your safety online. Let's look at some simple yet effective ways to protect yourself in the digital sphere.

Strong Passwords

In the online world, your password is like a key to your personal information. Creating strong, unique passwords for each online account is the first step towards digital safety. Use a mix of letters, numbers, and symbols to make your password hard to guess. Avoid using obvious information like your name, birth date, or simple sequences.

When creating passwords, avoid obvious choices like "123456" or "password." Instead, aim for complexity. A strong password should ideally be a mix of upper and lower-case letters, numbers, and symbols. For example, instead of "puppylove," consider "Pu99y!L0v3."

An effective practice is to use a phrase that means something to you, which can be easily remembered but hard for others to guess. For instance, "My son Sam loves 2 dogs!" can be turned into a password like "MsSl2d!"

Recognizing Email Scams

Scam emails or phishing attempts can sometimes find their way into your inbox, disguised as legitimate messages. Be wary of emails that ask for personal information, contain suspicious links, or have a sense of urgency. Remember, legitimate companies never ask for sensitive information via email. Also, have a safe friend or family member you can talk to about it before responding to any such emails regarding important matters.

Pay attention to the email's tone and content. Poor grammar, misspellings, or a lack of specific information can also be red flags. When in doubt, contact the organization directly using the official contact details listed on their website, not the information provided in the suspicious email.

Safe Online Shopping

Browsing through online stores, finding that perfect item, and making a purchase with just a few clicks can be an enjoyable experience. However, it's important to ensure your online shopping is secure.

Before making a purchase, check that the website address starts with "https." The "s" stands for secure, indicating that the site uses encryption to protect your information.

When it comes to payment, credit cards often offer better fraud protection than debit cards. Some online retailers and payment services offer their own security measures. For instance, PayPal conceals your credit card number from the seller.

Finally, always check your credit card statements for any unfamiliar transactions. If you spot something suspicious, report it immediately.

Safe Surfing

As you surf or search the internet, also be mindful of pop-up ads. If you are clicking too fast, you could end up caught in a virtual trap. Recently I was searching for an emotion wheel to share with someone. As I was clicking on the different images to see which one looked most similar to what they needed, I got caught. Caught in the web of a scammer disguised as the Virus protection app on my computer.

When it first came up, I turned off my computer and restarted it. No virus warning. I thought I was OK, but as soon as I opened the internet, it seemed to control my screen because of the unrelenting pop-up red flashing warnings. From my phone, I purchased a different antivirus protection. It installed and ran on my computer and said all clear, no threats. When I opened the internet, it happened all over again.

I spoke to my brother-in-law, and after I described what happened, he said to clear my browser history, delete the cookies, and restart the computer. Once I did this, everything was perfect. See, this was not a virus on my computer as it led me to believe. It was attached to the browser or web page I visited. I share this experience in hopes it will come to mind if it ever happens to someone you know and you can help them.

Privacy Settings

While the internet allows us to share and connect, it's crucial to control who sees what we share. Adjusting your privacy settings is like closing the curtains on your windows; you decide what to reveal and what to keep private.

Social media platforms and online accounts come with adjustable privacy settings, allowing you to control who sees your information and how they can interact with you. Regularly review and update these settings to protect your online privacy. You can often control who can see your posts, who can contact you, and what information is visible on your public profile.

Remember, the digital world is like any public space. While it offers numerous opportunities for learning, connection, and entertainment, it's important to ensure your safety and security. By taking these precautions, you can enjoy all the benefits of the digital world with peace of mind. So, set those strong passwords, keep an eye out for scams, shop safely, and manage your privacy settings. Your digital safety is in your hands, and with these tools, you're well-equipped to protect it.

As we wrap up this chapter, let's keep in mind that embracing technology doesn't mean compromising on safety. With strong passwords, awareness of email scams, safe online shopping practices, and proper privacy settings, we can enjoy the digital world confidently and securely. Now, let's look forward to the next chapter, where we'll explore another enriching facet of retirement life.

Chapter 9: Home Sweet Home: The Art of Living Well Indoors

"Retirement is the chapter of life where the canvas of our lives transforms into a gallery of indoor pursuits, a symphony of hobbies, and a sanctuary of contentment. Embrace the art of living well indoors, where every day is a masterpiece waiting to be created and enjoyed."

Picture this - you're lounging comfortably in your favorite armchair, a steaming cup of coffee by your side, and a fascinating book in your hands. The afternoon sun pours in through the window, casting a warm, inviting glow around the room. This is your sanctuary, your retreat, the place where you spend your retirement days. It's the place where you can explore new hobbies, entertain friends, and simply enjoy the pleasures of a well-lived life. In this chapter, we'll explore some engaging home-based activities that can enrich your retirement life right from the comfort of your home.

9.1 Home-Based Hobbies: Rediscovering Your Living Space

Indoor Gardening: A Touch of Green Indoors

You don't need a sprawling backyard or a sunny patio to enjoy the pleasures of gardening. Indoor gardening is like having a mini paradise right in your living room. It's about nurturing life, adding a touch of green to your space, and creating a tranquil environment to unwind.

You can start with easy-to-care-for plants like succulents, snake plants, or pothos. These plants not only purify the air but also add an aesthetic appeal to your home. All you need is a bright window, some pots, and a watering schedule. Remember, watching a plant grow can be a rewarding experience, a testament to your care and nurturing.

Home Cinema Nights: Bringing the Big Screen to Your Living Room

Who needs crowded movie theaters when you can enjoy a cinematic experience right at home? Home cinema nights are about popping some popcorn, dimming the lights, and getting lost in the world of movies.

You could host a weekly movie night where you and your friends take turns picking a movie. From timeless classics and inspiring documentaries to the latest blockbusters, the choices are endless. It's a fun way to experience the magic of cinema, share laughter, and create memorable evenings.

Book Clubs: A Literary Feast at Home

If you enjoy reading, why not share that joy with your friends? Hosting a book club at your home can be a delightful way to discuss favorite books, discover new authors, and engage in intellectual discussions.

You could choose a theme for each month, such as mystery novels, biographies, or award-winning books. The discussion could be paired with themed snacks or a potluck dinner, adding a social and culinary dimension to the literary feast. A book club is not just about reading; it's about sharing perspectives, broadening horizons, and creating a community of book lovers.

DIY Beauty Treatments: Spa Day at Home

Who says pampering needs to be expensive or outside your home? With DIY beauty treatments, you can enjoy a spa day right in your living room. It's about taking time to care for your body, to relax, and to enjoy some much-deserved pampering.

You could start with simple treatments like homemade face masks, sugar scrubs, or a relaxing foot soak. Invite some friends over for a spa day and turn it into a social event. It's a fun and affordable way to enjoy the spa experience with a dash of creativity and a lot of relaxation.

As we explore these home-based activities, let's remember that our homes are not just places where we live; they are spaces where we can learn, create, relax, and socialize. By exploring indoor gardening, home cinema nights, book clubs, and DIY beauty treatments, we can transform our homes into hubs of activity, creativity, and relaxation. So, let's get started on creating a living space that reflects our interests, caters to our hobbies, and enhances our retirement life.

9.2 Cooking and Baking: The Culinary Arts

Healthy Recipe Exploration

The kitchen, the heart of your home, is the perfect place to kick-start a nutritious adventure. With an abundance of wholesome recipes available online and in cookbooks, eating healthy has never been easier or tastier. Swap out processed foods for fresh ingredients, experiment with herbs and spices instead of relying on excess salt, and incorporate more fruits and vegetables into your meals. From vibrant salads and hearty soups to lean proteins and whole grains, there's a world of nourishing and delicious foods to explore. Each meal is an opportunity to fuel your body with the nutrients it needs while satisfying your taste buds.

Baking Bread and Pastries

The aroma of freshly baked bread wafting through your home is a sensory delight. Baking your own bread can be a therapeutic process, transforming simple ingredients into warm, fluffy loaves. Start with a basic white bread recipe, gradually venturing into whole wheat, sourdough, or even artisanal bread. The rhythmic kneading, the anticipation as the dough rises, and the satisfaction of tucking into your homemade bread, it's a wholesome and rewarding experience.

The world of baking doesn't stop at bread. Pastries, pies, cakes, and cookies are all delectable treats you can create in your own kitchen. Start simple, like a classic apple pie or chocolate chip cookies, gradually tackling more complex recipes. Baking can be quite a joy, a perfect blend of science and creativity, resulting in sweet (and savory) rewards.

International Cuisine Cooking

Retirement is a time to embrace new experiences, and that includes culinary adventures. Bring the world to your kitchen by trying your hand at international cuisine. Each country has its unique flavors and cooking techniques, from the creamy curries of India, the sushi of Japan, the pasta of Italy, to the tacos of Mexico.

Cooking dishes from around the world not only broadens your palate but also provides an understanding and appreciation for other cultures. So, dust off your passport and take your taste buds on a global tour, no luggage required.

Preserving and Canning

Preserving and canning is a time-honored tradition that allows you to enjoy seasonal fruits and vegetables all year round. Imagine opening a jar of homemade strawberry jam in the middle of winter or enjoying your own pickles with a cheese board. From jams, jellies, and pickles to canned fruits and vegetables, the options are endless.

Begin with something simple like a raspberry jam or pickled cucumbers. As you get the hang of the preserving and canning process, you can experiment with different recipes. It's a wonderful way to make the most of the season's bounty and a delightful addition to your pantry.

In conclusion, the kitchen is more than just a place to prepare meals. It's a playground for flavors, a canvas for culinary creativity, and a hub for nourishing your body and soul. Whether it's experimenting with healthy recipes, baking fresh bread, exploring international cuisine, or preserving seasonal produce, each activity adds a dash of flavor to your retirement life. So, put on your apron, fire up the stove, and let's cook up some great times in the kitchen.

9.3 Gardening: The Therapeutic Power of Nature

Flower Gardening: Cultivating Beauty

Imagine stepping outside to a riot of colors, your senses greeted by the intoxicating scent of blossoms. Flower gardening allows you to create your own personal oasis, a retreat from the everyday hustle and bustle. It's not just about having a pretty yard; it's about the joy of sowing a seed, watching it sprout and bloom into a gorgeous flower.

Starting a flower garden can be as simple as picking a sunny spot in your yard, preparing the soil, and planting your favorite flowers. You can choose annuals for a burst of color all summer or opt for perennials that will return year after year. From roses, tulips, and sunflowers to daisies, pansies, and petunias, your garden can be a canvas painted with nature's most vibrant hues.

Vegetable and Herb Gardening: Farm to Table

There's something incredibly satisfying about pulling a fresh carrot from your garden or snipping fresh herbs for your dinner.

Vegetable and herb gardening is like having a farmer's market right in your backyard. It's about the thrill of growing your own food, the satisfaction of self-reliance, and the enjoyment of unbeatable freshness.

You can start small with easy-to-grow veggies like lettuce, tomatoes, and bell peppers or herbs like basil, parsley, and mint. All you need is a sunny spot, good soil, and regular watering. As you gain confidence, you can expand your garden to include more varieties. Just imagine stepping outside and picking fresh produce for your meals. It doesn't get fresher than that!

Butterfly Gardens: Inviting Nature's Visitors

Picture a sunny afternoon, your garden alive with the fluttering of butterflies, their vivid wings adding a dash of magic to your garden. Creating a butterfly garden is about more than just aesthetics; it's about offering a habitat for these beautiful creatures and playing a part in your local ecosystem.

To attract butterflies, you'll need to plant nectar-rich flowers that they feed on. Marigolds, lavender, and butterfly bushes are all excellent choices. Remember, a butterfly garden is not just about the butterflies; it's about the joy of watching these beautiful creatures flit and flutter about, adding a touch of enchantment to your everyday life.

Container Gardening: Small Spaces, Big Impact

For those who don't have large yards, container gardening offers a fantastic way to indulge your green thumb. It's about making the most of your patio, balcony, or windowsill, transforming them into miniature gardens that pack a big punch.

Almost any plant can be grown in a container, from ornamental flowers and lush foliage to herbs, vegetables, and even small fruit trees. You can experiment with different containers, from traditional pots to creative options like tin cans, wooden crates, or even old boots. The key is to ensure good drainage, use quality potting soil, and provide the right amount of water and sunlight.

In essence, gardening in retirement is about nurturing life, whether it's a blooming flower, a ripening tomato, a fluttering butterfly, or a thriving container plant. It's about your connection with nature, the peace it brings, and the satisfaction of creating a living, breathing outdoor space. So, put on your gardening gloves, grab your trowel, and let's turn your garden into a haven of beauty, tranquility, and life's simple pleasures.

9.4 Home Improvement Projects: Enhancing Your Living Space

Painting and Wallpapering: A Fresh Coat of Inspiration

Imagine the walls of your home as a canvas, waiting for a touch of color or a pattern to bring it to life. Painting or wallpapering your rooms can dramatically transform your space, creating a new ambiance and reflecting your personality.

You could opt for calming blues for your bedroom, energizing yellows for your kitchen, or perhaps a sophisticated wallpaper pattern for your living room. Remember to prepare your walls properly before painting or wallpapering, removing old paint or wallpaper, filling in any holes, and ensuring the surface is clean and smooth. A weekend spent with a paintbrush or wallpaper in hand can result in a refreshing new look for your home.

Furniture Restoration: Breathing New Life into Old Pieces

Furniture restoration is like discovering a hidden treasure in your attic or basement. That old wooden chair or worn-out table has the potential to become a stylish piece for your home. All it needs is some care, creativity, and a bit of elbow grease.

Start by cleaning the piece and making any necessary repairs. Then, you can decide to refinish it with a fresh coat of paint or stain or perhaps upholster it with a new fabric. Furniture restoration not only gives a new lease of life to your old pieces but also adds a personal touch to your home décor.

Organizing and Decluttering: A Place for Everything

A well-organized home is a joy to live in. Everything has its place, and you can easily find what you need. Start by sorting through your belongings, deciding what to keep, what to donate, and what to throw away.

Next, organize what's left in a way that makes sense to you. You might use storage boxes, shelves, or closet organizers to keep everything tidy. Remember, the goal of organizing isn't just to make your space look neat; it's to make your life easier and more efficient.

DIY Decor Projects: Your Home, Your Masterpiece

DIY decor projects are like adding your signature to your living space. It could be a hand-painted vase, a homemade wreath for your front door, or a photo collage on your wall. These projects not only add a personal touch to your home but also provide a satisfying and creative pastime.

You can find numerous DIY decor ideas and tutorials online, suitable for various skill levels. So, gather your supplies, roll up your sleeves, and let your creativity flow. Each project you complete adds a piece of you to your home.

Creating a Home Gym or Art Studio: Dedicated Spaces for Your Passions

Why not dedicate a space in your home for your hobbies and interests? A spare room, a corner of your living room, or even a part of your garage can become a home gym or an art studio.

For a home gym, you might invest in some basic equipment like weights, resistance bands, and a yoga mat. If art is your passion, your studio could have an easel, storage for your art supplies and good lighting. These dedicated spaces not only make it easier to engage in your favorite activities but also serve as a constant reminder to make time for what you love.

In the end, enhancing your living space is about creating a home that reflects you - your tastes, your interests, and your lifestyle. It's about making your home not just a place to live but a place to thrive in your retirement years. So, pick up that paintbrush, restore that old chair, organize your space, craft that decor item, and create that special corner for your hobbies. Your home is your canvas - make it a masterpiece of comfort, joy, and personal expression.

CHAPTER 10: NAVIGATING FINANCES IN YOUR GOLDEN YEARS

"Let's ensure our financial ship is sturdy, our sails set toward security, and our voyage through retirement smooth and fulfilling." - Lorie Eubank

Imagine standing atop a mountain, breathing in the fresh air, gazing at the stunning scenery below. Now, imagine reaching this peak not by helicopter but by a grueling hike. The panoramic view is the same, but the sense of achievement is incomparable. This is what financial planning in retirement is all about. It's not just about maintaining a lifestyle; it's about the satisfaction of managing your finances effectively, the peace of mind that comes with financial stability, and the freedom to enjoy your retirement years without financial stress. Let's get started on this rewarding hike.

10.1 Importance of Financial Health in Retirement

A sturdy house requires a solid foundation. Similarly, a fulfilling retirement life is built on the bedrock of financial health. Good financial health ensures that you can maintain your lifestyle, tackle unexpected expenses, and even indulge in your dreams and passions. Here are some factors that make financial health crucial during retirement:

Longevity and Inflation

Today, thanks to advancements in healthcare, we're living longer than ever before. While this is certainly a cause for celebration, it also means that your retirement savings need to last longer.

In addition, inflation is like a slow leak in a tire. Over time, it erodes the value of your money. What seems like a comfortable nest egg today may not have the same purchasing power a decade from now. Therefore, planning for longevity and inflation is like patching that leak, ensuring a smooth and worry-free ride through retirement.

Medical and Health Care Costs

As we age, medical and healthcare costs tend to rise. Regular check-ups, prescription medications, or even a sudden health issue can lead to significant expenses.

Consider this: You've been an avid gardener all your life. One day, while pruning your rose bushes, you slip and fall, resulting in a fractured wrist. Besides the immediate medical costs, there might be follow-up visits, physical therapy sessions, and even home care costs. Adequate financial planning can act as a safety net, protecting you from the financial impact of such unforeseen health issues.

Lifestyle Maintenance

Retirement is a time to enjoy the fruits of years of hard work. Whether it's traveling, pursuing hobbies, or simply enjoying leisure time with family and friends, maintaining your lifestyle plays a significant role in your happiness and satisfaction during retirement.

Picture this: You've always dreamed of visiting the cherry blossom festival in Japan. You've imagined walking under the beautiful Sakura trees, their pink blossoms creating a mesmerizing canopy. Good financial health can turn such dreams into reality. It ensures that your retirement years are not just about survival but about enjoyment, fulfillment, and making beautiful memories.

In conclusion, financial health in retirement is like a reliable compass. It guides you through the ups and downs, the twists and turns of your retirement journey. It provides a sense of direction, a sense of security, and, most importantly, a sense of freedom. So, let's equip ourselves with this compass and set forth on an adventure of financial planning and management in retirement. After all, every great adventure starts with a single step.

10.2 Budgeting for a Comfortable Life

How do you envision your retirement? Perhaps a quiet morning with a hot cup of tea, reading the latest best-seller. Or maybe an afternoon spent in the pottery class you've always wanted to take. Could it be a spontaneous road trip with old friends? All these delightful experiences share a common thread - they are influenced by your financial health. Hence, budgeting is not a restriction on your spending but a plan that enables you to enjoy your retirement to its fullest.

Fixed and Variable Expenses

In the grand tapestry of retirement budgeting, understanding your expenses is akin to knowing the threads you have at your disposal. Expenses typically fall into two categories - fixed and variable.

Fixed expenses are the regularly recurring costs that remain relatively stable over time. These would include rent or mortgage payments, utilities, insurance premiums, and any other established monthly costs. These are akin to the warp threads in your tapestry - they form the backbone of your budget.

Variable expenses, on the other hand, tend to fluctuate from month to month. These could include groceries, dining out, hobbies, travel, and personal care. Much like the weft threads, these expenses weave through your budget, adding color and texture to your retirement life.

Start by listing down all your expenses, both fixed and variable. For accuracy, refer to bank statements, receipts, bills, and credit card statements from the past few months. This will give you a clear picture of where your money is going and help you plan your budget effectively.

Emergency Fund

In the unpredictable dance of life, an emergency fund is your safety net. It's the financial cushion that softens the impact of unexpected expenses, such as home repairs, medical bills, or sudden travel.

How much should you set aside for emergencies? A general rule of thumb is to have enough to cover three to six months' worth of living expenses. Of course, this would vary depending on your lifestyle, health, and risk tolerance.

Remember, an emergency fund is not built overnight. Start small and aim to contribute regularly until you reach your goal. Knowing you have a safety net can provide peace of mind and financial security in your retirement years.

Leisure and Travel Budget

Retirement is your well-earned break, a time to indulge in hobbies, travel, and leisure activities. Allocating a part of your budget for leisure and travel ensures that you can enjoy these golden years without financial stress.

How much should you budget for leisure? This depends on your interests, health, and of course, your overall budget. If you're a travel enthusiast, you might choose to allocate a larger portion to your travel fund. If you're a hobbyist, your leisure budget might include art supplies, gardening tools, or perhaps photography equipment.

When budgeting for leisure, remember to factor in all costs. For instance, a vacation budget should include not just transportation and accommodation but also meals, sightseeing, shopping, and even travel insurance.

In essence, a well-planned budget is like a roadmap to a fulfilling retirement. It helps you navigate your expenses, prepare for emergencies, and enjoy your leisure time without financial worries. So, take the reins of your financial health, plan your budget, and look forward to a comfortable and enjoyable retirement life.

10.3 Investment Tips for Seniors

Picture yourself as a seasoned gardener, tending to a variety of plants in your garden. Each plant represents a different investment. The diversity not only adds beauty to your garden but also ensures that a failure of one plant doesn't ruin your entire garden. This is the essence of a diversification strategy in investing. Ask trusted family or friends to help you connect with a reliable Retirement Coach or Financial Adviser.

Diversification Strategy

Investing in a mix of assets is like planting a variety of seeds in your financial garden. Some investments will grow steadily over time, while others may offer higher returns but come with greater risks. The idea is to balance the risk and reward by spreading investments across different asset classes such as stocks, bonds, and real estate.

Just as a gardener knows that not all seeds will sprout, an investor understands that not all investments will yield high returns. However, a diversified portfolio can help minimize losses, as poor performance by one investment can be offset by strong performance by others.

Risk Tolerance Assessment

Just as every gardener has a different tolerance for dealing with weeds and pests, every investor has a different tolerance for risk. Risk tolerance refers to your ability and willingness to lose some or all of your original investment in exchange for greater potential returns.

An investor with a high-risk tolerance might have a larger portion of their portfolio invested in stocks, which can be volatile but offer higher potential returns. On the other hand, an investor with a low-risk tolerance might prefer bonds or money market funds, which offer lower returns but are less volatile.

Understanding your risk tolerance can guide you in selecting the right mix of investments to meet your financial goals and sleep comfortably at night.

Bonds and Fixed Income Securities

In the diverse garden of investments, bonds and other fixed-income securities are like sturdy trees that provide steady, reliable growth. When you purchase a bond, you're essentially lending money to an entity (like a corporation or government) in exchange for periodic interest payments and the return of the bond's face value when it matures.

Bonds can be a good choice for retirees as they provide regular income and are generally less risky than stocks. However, they're not completely risk-free. The issuer of the bond could default on their payments, or rising interest rates could make existing bonds less attractive.

Real Estate Investment Trusts

Imagine owning a piece of a shopping mall, an office building, or a hotel. Real Estate Investment Trusts (REITs) make this possible. REITs are companies that own, operate, or finance income-generating real estate. When you invest in a REIT, you're buying shares of that company and can profit from its earnings.

REITs can offer a way to invest in real estate without the need to buy or manage properties. They can provide a steady income stream, making them an attractive option for retirees. However, like any investment, they come with risks, including real estate market fluctuations and interest rate risks.

Investments are like seeds in your financial garden. With careful planning, regular care, and a bit of patience, they can grow into a thriving financial future. So, diversify your portfolio, assess your risk tolerance, consider bonds and REITs, and watch your retirement savings flourish. Happy gardening!

10.4 Estate Planning: Ensuring Your Legacy

Estate planning is like leaving a trail of breadcrumbs for your loved ones. It might not sound like the most exciting part of retirement planning, but it's undoubtedly one of the most crucial. It's about making decisions today that will provide clear guidance and ease the emotional and financial burden on your loved ones in the future.

Will and Testament

Think of a Will as a detailed roadmap you're leaving behind, guiding your loved ones through what can be a challenging journey. A Will is a legal document that spells out your wishes regarding the distribution of your assets and the care of any minor children.

Creating a Will is about putting pen to paper and detailing how you'd like your assets to be distributed. It's about eliminating guesswork and potential conflicts among your heirs. It's about ensuring your legacy is passed on in the way you intended.

Trust Funds

A Trust Fund, on the other hand, is like a treasure chest that you fill and leave behind for your heirs. It's a legal entity that holds and manages your assets for the benefit of specific individuals or organizations.

Establishing a Trust Fund can provide you with a certain level of control over how your assets are used even after you're gone. For instance, you can stipulate that the funds be used solely for the education of your grandchildren or the support of a beloved charity.

Power of Attorney

Appointing a Power of Attorney is like nominating a trusted co-pilot. It's a legal process where you grant a trusted individual the authority to make decisions on your behalf if you become unable to do so.

The person you appoint, known as an attorney-in-fact, can be granted authority over financial matters, legal issues, or health-related decisions. It's a role of significant responsibility, so it's crucial to appoint someone you trust implicitly.

Advance Health Care Directive

An Advance Health Care Directive, also known as a living will, is like a beacon in the fog. It's a document that outlines your wishes regarding your medical treatment if you're unable to communicate them yourself.

Creating an Advance Health Care Directive is about making challenging decisions in advance, sparing your loved ones from having to make them in a crisis. It's about making your values and preferences known, ensuring that your treatment aligns with your wishes, even if you can't express them.

In the grand scheme of retirement planning, estate planning is a pivotal piece of the puzzle. It's about tying up loose ends, providing guidance, and ensuring your legacy lives on in the way you intended. It's not just about the legalities; it's about the peace of mind that comes from knowing you've done all you can to ease the path for your loved ones. So, draft that Will, set up that Trust Fund, appoint that Power of Attorney, and create that Advance Health Care Directive. It's your legacy; let it be a testament to your life, your values, and your love for your dear ones.

As we close this chapter, we realize that while retirement involves a shift in lifestyle, it also presents an opportunity to plan and manage our financial resources wisely. The retirement years can be filled with joy, peace, and fulfillment when underpinned by sound financial planning. With this in mind, let's step into the next chapter, where we will explore the various housing options in retirement and how these can impact our lifestyle and finances.

Chapter 11: Housing in Retirement: Your Comfort, Your Choice

"Housing in retirement is not just about a place to live; it's about creating the haven of comfort and choice where you can savor the joys of this new chapter on your terms."

Picture this: A gentle breeze rustling through the leaves, a cozy armchair by the window, the familiar aroma of your morning coffee. This is home, the space where you unwind, create memories and live out your golden years. But what makes a house a home in retirement? Is it the number of rooms, the proximity to family, the accessibility features, or perhaps, a combination of all these factors? In this chapter, we'll explore how to evaluate your housing needs in retirement, ensuring your home is not just a dwelling but a haven of comfort, convenience, and joy.

Home, they say, is where the heart is. But when it comes to retirement, the heart needs a bit of practicality too. As we age, our housing needs evolve. The bustling family home might seem too large, the stairs might seem daunting, and the maintenance might feel overwhelming. On the other hand, the familiar neighborhood, the proximity to friends and family, the emotional attachment to the house, all these factors tug at the heartstrings, making the decision complex. Let's break it down and examine some key factors to consider while evaluating your housing needs.

11.1 Evaluating Your Housing Needs

Space Requirements

Think of your living space as a canvas. The size of the canvas should not constrict your lifestyle; instead, it should provide ample room for your daily activities, hobbies, and social gatherings.

Too large a house can become a burden with time, considering the cleaning, maintenance, and higher utility bills. On the other hand, too small a space can feel cramped and limit your activities. Evaluate your current usage of space. Do you use all the rooms in your house, or do certain areas remain closed off, collecting dust? Perhaps you could do with fewer rooms but desire a larger kitchen or a spacious patio.

Consider your future needs as well. If you're planning to pursue a hobby that requires space, like painting or woodworking, ensure you have a dedicated area for it. If you're expecting frequent visits from family and friends, an extra guest room could be beneficial.

Accessibility Features

Remember, your home should cater to you, not the other way around. As we age, certain tasks can become challenging. An accessible home can make daily routines safer and more comfortable, giving you the confidence to live independently.

Some features to consider are single-floor living, wide doorways for potential wheelchair access, a step-in shower, and grab bars in the bathroom. The goal is to create an environment that minimizes the risk of falls and makes navigation easy.

While some homes might already include these features, others might require modifications. Consider the feasibility of these changes, the associated costs, and the value they add to your quality of life.

Proximity to Family and Services

Location is like the soil in which your home is rooted. It should provide nourishment in the form of access to essential services and emotional connection through proximity to loved ones.

How close do you want to be to your family and friends? Would you prefer to live in the same neighborhood or the same city?

Or perhaps, you're okay with living a flight away, given there are reliable transport options.

Access to medical facilities is another crucial factor, especially if you have ongoing health conditions. The proximity to shopping centers, recreational facilities, and public transport also adds to the convenience.

Remember, retirement is a new beginning, a stage of life that brings with it changes and choices. Choosing the right home, a space that accommodates your needs, enhances your comfort, and resonates with your lifestyle, is a significant decision in this journey. So, take your time, weigh the pros and cons, and listen to both your heart and your mind. After all, home is more than just a place to live; it's the backdrop of your retirement life, the stage where the beautiful play of your golden years unfolds.

11.2 Understanding Your Options: From Downsizing to Active Adult Communities

Condominiums and Townhouses: Easy Living in Compact Spaces

Imagine swapping the sprawling lawns and lengthy maintenance of a house for the compact, easy-to-manage space of a condo or townhouse. Condominiums and townhouses offer the comfort of a home without the responsibilities of extensive upkeep.

Usually located in urban or suburban areas, they provide easy access to amenities and community activities.

In a condominium, you own your unit and share common areas with other residents. This may include amenities like swimming pools, gyms, and communal spaces. Typically, a homeowners association takes care of the maintenance and repair of these shared spaces, covered by your association fees. This leaves you more time to enjoy your retirement activities and less time worrying about property upkeep.

Townhouses, on the other hand, are multi-floor homes connected in a row. They offer more privacy than condos and often come with a small yard. Like condos, townhouses usually have an association that takes care of common areas.

Living in a condo or townhouse can foster a sense of community, with neighbors close by and communal activities. However, it's important to consider the rules and regulations of the homeowners association, the association fees, and the level of privacy.

Senior Co-housing: Community Living with Independence

How about living in a community where you share not only spaces but also experiences, responsibilities, and camaraderie with fellow seniors? Senior co-housing is a concept that brings together a group of seniors to live in individual homes within a shared property.

In senior co-housing, residents have their private residences but also share common facilities like a dining area, gardens, and recreational spaces. The residents manage the community, make decisions collectively, and often share meals and activities. This model combines the advantages of private housing with the benefits of communal living, fostering social connections and mutual support while respecting individual independence.

Co-housing can be a rewarding option for those who enjoy community living, and shared responsibilities, and are comfortable with consensus decision-making. It's crucial to understand the dynamics of the co-housing community, the financial implications, and the level of commitment required.

Assisted Living Facilities: Supportive Living with Care

If you're considering a living option that combines independence with support for daily living activities, an assisted living facility could be the answer. Assisted living facilities offer a residential setting with personal care services, meals, and recreational activities.

Residents have their apartments or rooms and share common areas. They receive assistance with daily activities like bathing, dressing, medication management, and transportation. Meals are usually served in a communal dining area, and a variety of social and recreational activities are organized for residents.

Assisted living can be a suitable choice for those who need some assistance with daily activities but do not require the intensive care of a nursing home. As this is a significant lifestyle change, it's important to consider the quality of care, the range of services, the environment, and the costs involved.

11.3 Making Your Home Age-Friendly

Home Safety Modifications

The home you've grown to love over the years might need a few tweaks to keep up with your evolving needs in retirement. Think of these modifications as friendly adaptations that make your house more accommodating and comfortable.

Let's start with the stairs, often a significant concern for seniors. Installing handrails on both sides can provide support and balance. If your bedroom is upstairs, consider converting a downstairs room into a bedroom to avoid frequent stair navigation.

Bathrooms can be tricky too. Installing grab bars near the toilet and in the shower can provide added stability. Non-slip mats can prevent slips and falls, while a shower seat can make bathing safer and more comfortable.

In the kitchen, rearranging your items can make a world of difference. Keep frequently used items in easily accessible lower cabinets. If you need to use a step stool for higher shelves, ensure it's sturdy and has a handrail.

Remember, these modifications aren't concessions but thoughtful changes to make your home safer and more comfortable.

Smart Home Technology for Seniors

In this digital age, technology has snuck into our homes, making life more convenient and efficient. For seniors, smart home technology can offer added safety, automation, and even companionship.

Voice-controlled devices, like Amazon Alexa or Google Home, can perform a myriad of tasks. They can play your favorite music, remind you of medication times, or even tell you a joke when you need a chuckle.

Smart lighting systems can be programmed to turn on or off at certain times or controlled remotely. No more fumbling for light switches in the dark.

Then there are smart home security systems. Door sensors, security cameras, and alarm systems can provide peace of mind, keeping you informed about who's at the door or any unusual activity.

While these gadgets may seem intimidating at first, remember that they are designed to be user-friendly. Take one step at a time, and slowly, you'll find these smart devices becoming your friendly home assistants.

Gardening and Outdoor Spaces

The outdoors, the symphony of birdsong, the fragrance of fresh blooms, and the dance of butterflies have a charm of their own. Making your garden or outdoor space senior-friendly means you can enjoy Mother Nature's show in comfort and safety.

Start with garden maintenance. Opt for low-maintenance plants that require less watering and pruning. Raised garden beds or potted plants can be easier on the back as they reduce the need to bend.

Think about installing a comfortable bench or swing where you can sit and enjoy the outdoors. Ensure pathways are smooth and even to prevent tripping, and consider installing outdoor lighting for visibility in the evenings.

For those who love gardening, consider adaptive gardening tools. They are designed to reduce strain on the body and make gardening tasks easier.

Your garden or outdoor space is an extension of your home, a personal oasis. With a few modifications, it can become a haven where you can bask in the sun, enjoy the fresh air, and take delight in the natural beauty around you.

11.4 When Home is on the Move: The RV Lifestyle

Choosing the Right RV

Picture your mornings, the sunlight streaming through the window, the scent of fresh coffee wafting through the air, and the open road beckoning you to new adventures. This is the RV lifestyle, a blend of comfort, freedom, and exploration. The first step in embracing this lifestyle is selecting the right RV.

RVs, short for Recreational Vehicles, are your home on wheels. They vary in size, features, and price, catering to diverse needs and budgets. Class A motorhomes are the largest, offering luxury accommodations and amenities. Class B motorhomes, also known as campervans, are smaller but offer efficient use of space and ease of driving. Class C motorhomes are a blend of the two, offering more space than campervans without the hefty size of Class A motorhomes.

Consider your travel plans, the number of people traveling with you, your budget, and your comfort preferences when choosing an RV. Remember, the right RV is one that turns the open road into a homely path.

RV Parks and Communities

RV Parks are like neighborhoods on the go, offering a space to park your RV, essential amenities, and a sense of community. These parks usually provide electric, water, and sewer hookups, along with facilities like laundry, restrooms, Wi-Fi, and sometimes even a swimming pool or a clubhouse.

RV communities, on the other hand, are designed for longer stays. They offer larger lots, more amenities, and organized social activities. Some are age-restricted, catering specifically to the 55+ demographic, fostering a community of like-minded, similarly aged individuals.

Choosing the right RV park or community depends on your needs, preferences, and the duration of your stay. It's about finding a place that offers the conveniences you need, the ambiance you enjoy, and the community you feel at home with.

Travel Planning and Budgeting

Stepping into the RV lifestyle is like charting your own course on the map of retirement. Travel planning involves deciding your destinations, the routes you'll take, the sights you want to see, and the time you want to spend at each location. Be sure to consider the weather, the driving conditions, and the availability of RV parks at your chosen destinations.

Budgeting, an inseparable companion of planning, ensures your RV adventures are enjoyable without straining your finances. Consider the cost of fuel, campground fees, meals, sightseeing, and unexpected expenses like repairs or maintenance.

Traveling in an RV doesn't mean you have to cook all your meals. Plan for dining out or takeaway meals now and then. Remember, the local cuisine is an integral part of the travel experience.

In the grand scheme of retirement living, the RV lifestyle offers an alternative path. It combines the comforts of home with the thrill of travel, the familiarity of a community with the excitement of new encounters. It's about steering your retirement life in the direction of your dreams, one mile at a time. So, choose your RV, find your community, plan your travels, and let the road ahead be a testament to your adventurous spirit and your love for life.

As the sun sets on this chapter, let's carry forward the insights, ideas, and inspirations into the next exciting phase of our retirement journey. A new dawn awaits us, bringing new topics to explore, new ideas to embrace, and new paths to tread on our quest to make the most of our golden years. So, buckle up, dear reader; the journey continues.

Chapter 12: Embracing the Encore: Crafting Your Post-Retirement Career

"Retirement is not the end of your career; it's the beginning of your encore, a chance to craft a new career that aligns with your passions, talents, and dreams."

Have you ever watched an exciting movie, only to be left wanting more when the credits roll? That's where sequels come in, offering an extension of the story, a fresh perspective, and an encore. Apply this cinematic metaphor to your career, and you've got the concept of an encore career. It's not about rehashing the same plot but embarking on a new narrative that's driven by passion, purpose, and the desire for continued growth.

In this chapter, we'll explore the concept of the encore career, the various forms it can take, and how it can add a new dimension to your retirement life. Remember, retirement isn't the end credits of your professional life; it's the start of an exciting sequel, a chance to continue contributing, learning, and growing.

12.1 Defining the Encore Career

Part-time Work: The Best of Both Worlds

Let's start with part-time work. Imagine spending a few hours each day doing something you enjoy and getting paid for it. That's the beauty of part-time work in retirement. It offers the perfect balance between work and leisure, allowing you to stay engaged in the workforce without the stress of a full-time job.

You could choose to work part-time in your pre-retirement field, capitalizing on your experience and skills. Alternatively, you could explore a completely different industry that interests you. It could be anything from working at a local library, tutoring students in your favorite subject, or even helping out at a neighborhood coffee shop. The key is to find something that you enjoy, offers a sense of fulfillment, and aligns with your retirement lifestyle.

Consulting or Freelancing: Leverage Your Expertise

Have you spent years honing your skills and building expertise in a particular field? Why not put that to good use in your retirement? Consulting or freelancing allows you to leverage your knowledge and experience, helping others while earning an income.

For example, if you've spent your career in marketing, you could offer consulting services to startups needing marketing strategies. If you're a retired teacher, you could offer private tutoring or create online courses. The possibilities are as varied as your skills and experiences.

The flexibility of consulting or freelancing can be a significant advantage in retirement. You can choose the projects you take on, work at your own pace, and often set your own rates. It's a way to stay connected with your professional field while enjoying the freedom and flexibility of retirement.

Starting a Business: Ignite Your Entrepreneurial Spirit

Have you ever dreamed of starting your own business? Retirement could be the perfect time to ignite your entrepreneurial spirit. Maybe you have a unique business idea, a product you want to develop, or a service you want to offer. Starting a business in retirement can be a fulfilling endeavor that combines creativity, strategy, and hard work.

Consider turning a hobby into a business. If you love gardening, you could start a small nursery or offer gardening classes. If you're a whiz in the kitchen, consider starting a catering service or selling homemade goods. The key is to choose a business idea that excites you, aligns with your skills, and has potential in the market.

Starting a business requires planning, financial investment, and a lot of determination. But, with the right idea and the right approach, it can add a whole new level of excitement and purpose to your retirement life.

In conclusion, an encore career in retirement is about blending passion, experience, and the desire for continued growth. Whether it's part-time work, consulting, freelancing, or starting a business, the encore stage can be a rewarding extension of your professional life. It's about defining success in your own terms, contributing in your unique way, and writing a sequel that's as compelling as the original story. After all, the show isn't over until the final curtain call, and in your retirement, you're just getting ready for the encore.

12.2 Reaping the Rewards: The Upsides of Working in Retirement

In the vibrant tapestry of retirement life, an encore career can add a unique blend of colors. These are the colors of financial stability, intellectual engagement, and social connection. Each shade contributes to enhancing the quality of your retirement, making it as enriching as it is enjoyable. Let's take a closer look at these benefits and how they can paint a beautiful picture of your golden years.

Financial Stability: Keeping the Coffers Full

Think of your financial stability as a well-stocked pantry. It's the assurance that you have enough provisions to whip up a hearty meal anytime. An encore career, in this context, is like a flourishing vegetable garden, supplementing your pantry with fresh produce.

Working in retirement can provide an additional source of income, supplementing your savings, pension, or Social Security benefits. It's not just about money for daily expenses but also about having the financial freedom to indulge in your interests, travel, or spoil your grandkids. It can also provide a buffer against unforeseen expenses, ensuring your retirement nest egg lasts longer.

Moreover, continuing to earn a paycheck can offer a sense of financial independence. It's the satisfaction of knowing that you're not entirely reliant on your savings or the government for your financial needs.

Mental Stimulation: Keeping the Mind Sharp

Now, imagine your mind as a puzzle, one that thrives on challenges, problem-solving, and continuous learning. An encore career can be the missing piece that keeps this puzzle complete and vibrant.

Staying mentally active is crucial for cognitive health as we age. Work, regardless of the form it takes, provides cognitive stimulation. It keeps you thinking, learning, and problem-solving. Whether you're strategizing for a business, learning new software, or navigating the challenges of part-time work, you're exercising your brain, keeping it fit and agile.

An encore career can also offer a sense of purpose, a reason to get up every morning with a goal in mind. It can provide structure to your days, something that many people miss in the unstructured nature of retirement.

Social Interaction: Creating Connections

Lastly, let's consider the vibrant colors of social interaction in our retirement tapestry. Working in retirement can offer ample opportunities to socialize, network, and build meaningful relationships.

Workplaces, whether physical or virtual, are social hubs. They offer a sense of community, a sense of belonging. Through your encore career, you can meet people of different ages, backgrounds, and perspectives. You can engage in stimulating conversations, share ideas, and even form friendships. For many, coworkers become an extended family, providing support, camaraderie, and a sense of belonging.

Moreover, an encore career can help maintain your professional identity. It allows you to continue contributing to your field, stay updated with industry trends, and maintain your professional networks.

In essence, an encore career can add a unique blend of financial stability, mental stimulation, and social interaction to your retirement life. It can enhance your golden years, making them not just comfortable but also fulfilling, engaging, and socially connected. So, as you navigate your retirement, consider the vibrant colors an encore career can add to your life's tapestry. After all, every artist knows that the right blend of colors can turn a blank canvas into a masterpiece.

12.3 Finding Your Encore Career

Skills and Passion Assessment

A fascinating aspect of retirement is the opportunity to reflect, reassess, and recalibrate. When it comes to your encore career, this process begins with a thorough evaluation of your skills and passions.

Begin by taking inventory of your abilities. What are you good at? This could include hard skills, like proficiency in a foreign language or computer programming, and soft skills, like communication, leadership, or problem-solving. Don't limit yourself to skills you've used in your previous career. Think broadly about abilities you've developed through hobbies, volunteer work, or even life experiences.

Next, consider your passions. What activities make you lose track of time? What causes ignite a spark in you? What dreams have you harbored that you now have the time and freedom to pursue? This could be anything from painting, teaching, gardening to helping underprivileged kids, saving the environment, or advocating for animal rights.

Remember, your encore career should not be a mere continuation of your prior work life but an alignment of your skills and passions. It's about creating a synergy between what you're good at and what you love doing, ultimately leading to a career that offers satisfaction, fulfillment, and joy.

Networking and Job Search

With a clear understanding of your skills and passions, you're ready to venture into the job market. Networking and job search are like two sides of the same coin, each playing a crucial role in landing your ideal encore career.

Networking is about cultivating relationships and creating a support system in your professional world. Reach out to former colleagues, attend industry events, participate in online forums, or join local clubs related to your field of interest. Networking not only opens doors to job opportunities but also provides support, advice, and camaraderie on your encore career journey.

Job search, on the other hand, is about actively seeking out opportunities that match your skills and passions. Traditional job search methods like newspaper ads and employment agencies still work, but don't overlook the power of the internet. Online job portals, company websites, and professional networking sites like LinkedIn can be effective tools in your job search arsenal.

When exploring job opportunities, consider not just the role and the pay but also the work culture, flexibility, and learning opportunities. Your encore career should align with your retirement lifestyle, not disrupt it.

Training and Education Opportunities

Learning is a lifelong endeavor, and retirement is no exception. As you gear up for your encore career, consider if there are any skills you need to brush up on or new ones you wish to acquire.

Thanks to technology, there are myriad ways to pursue training and education from the comfort of your home. Online courses, webinars, and workshops offer flexible learning options in a wide range of subjects. Local community colleges and adult education centers also offer courses tailored for seniors.

If your encore career involves starting a business, you might want to take a course in entrepreneurship or small business management. If you're interested in teaching, a course in instructional strategies could be beneficial. If technology intimidates you, consider a basic computer course.

Remember, pursuing training and education not only enhances your skills but also boosts your confidence. It's a testament to your commitment to continuous growth and adaptability. It's a reminder that no matter your age, you can always learn something new, take on a challenge, and embrace the exciting opportunities that life presents.

In the end, finding your encore career is about introspection, exploration, and education. It's about aligning your skills and passions, reaching out to your network, seeking out opportunities, and embracing lifelong learning. It's about crafting a career that adds meaning, fulfillment, and an extra dose of excitement to your retirement life. So, take that first step, seize the day, and make your encore career a performance to remember.

12.4 Balancing Work and Leisure in Retirement

Time Management: The Symphony of Your Day

Imagine your day as a symphony, a melodic arrangement of work, leisure, and rest. The art of time management in retirement is about directing this symphony, ensuring a harmonious balance of activities that contribute to a fulfilling day.

Start by creating a flexible daily schedule. This isn't about rigid time blocks but a general outline of how you'd like your day to unfold. You might allot certain hours for work, carve out time for leisure activities, and ensure ample time for relaxation and self-care.

Consider your energy patterns. If you're a morning person, schedule your work hours during the morning when your energy and concentration levels are high. Reserve the afternoon for lighter activities or hobbies. If you're a night owl, adjust your schedule accordingly.

Remember, retirement is your time to shine, devoid of the 9 to 5 constraints. It's about managing your time in a way that aligns with your lifestyle and preferences and encore career commitments.

Work-Life Balance: The Dance of Your Golden Years

If time management is the symphony of your day, work-life balance is the dance of your retirement life. It's about moving gracefully between professional commitments and personal pursuits, ensuring neither overwhelms the other.

Working in retirement isn't about replicating the stress or workload of your pre-retirement career. It's about creating a career that complements your retirement lifestyle, not competing with it. Design your work commitments in a way that leaves ample time for leisure, relaxation, social activities, and spontaneous adventures.

Remember, the beauty of an encore career lies in its flexibility. You have the freedom to choose how much you work and when. It's about creating a rhythm that brings joy, fulfillment, and a sense of balance to your life.

Health and Wellness Prioritization: The Lifeline of Your Retirement

In the vibrant canvas of retirement, health, and wellness are the lifelines that add vitality to every stroke. Prioritizing your health and wellness is about ensuring these lifelines remain strong and vibrant, supporting you in all your endeavors.

Incorporate regular exercise into your daily routine. It could be a brisk morning walk, a yoga session, or a dance class. Regular physical activity not only keeps you fit but also boosts your mood and energy levels.

Mindful eating is another crucial aspect. Nourish your body with a balanced diet rich in fruits, vegetables, lean proteins, and whole grains. Stay hydrated and limit the intake of processed foods and sugar.

Don't forget about your mental and emotional health. Cultivate mindfulness through meditation or breathing exercises. Engage in activities that bring you joy and relaxation. Stay socially connected, whether it's through work, family gatherings, or community activities.

Lastly, ensure regular health check-ups and listen to your body. If you feel tired or overwhelmed, take a break. Your health and wellness are not just the lifelines of your retirement; they're the foundation of a fulfilling encore career and a vibrant retirement life.

So here you are, standing at the threshold of an exciting new phase. Retirement isn't about fading into the sunset; it's about rising to a new dawn of opportunities, experiences, and adventures. With an encore career, you're not just working; you're crafting a lifestyle that's brimming with passion, purpose, and potential. So, step forward with confidence, embrace the dance of work and leisure, and let the symphony of your retirement life play its melodious tune. Let's look forward to the next chapter, where we'll explore another enriching facet of retirement life.

Conclusion: Reflecting on Your Retirement Journey

Well, here we are, my friend. We've reached the end of this journey together, but as they say, every end is just a new beginning. Looking back, we've navigated through the myths and realities of retirement, explored exciting activities, and even painted the canvas of our golden years with an encore career. We've learned to embrace change as an integral part of this journey and discovered that retirement is not the end, but a delightful bend in the road of life.

Embracing the Future: Your Retirement, Your Way

As we move forward, remember that your retirement is yours to shape, like a potter at the wheel. Whether you choose to explore the world in an RV, start a small business, or simply enjoy the tranquility of your garden, the choice is yours. Just as each sunrise brings a new day, each day of your retirement brings new possibilities. Embrace them, savor them, and weave them into the rich tapestry of your retirement life.

Celebrating Your Golden Years: Embrace Life's New Chapter

Your retirement years are a time to celebrate, a time to reflect on your achievements and look forward to new adventures. It's a time to discover new interests, make new friendships, and create lasting memories. Remember, each wrinkle is a testament to laughter shared, challenges overcome, and lessons learned. So, wear them as badges of honor as you dance into this new chapter of life.

Final Thoughts: The Journey Continues

As we wrap up this guide, remember that the journey continues. Retirement is not a destination but a voyage of discovery, growth, and fulfillment. Even as we turn the last page of this book, remember that you're just turning the first page of your exciting retirement story.

I hope this guide has been a helpful companion, shedding light on the path and igniting ideas for your retirement years. I wish you joy, health, and a sense of wonder as you embark on this exciting journey. Remember, my friend, retirement is not the sunset of life but a beautiful sunrise waiting to illuminate your path. Embrace it, live it, and make every moment count.

Here's to the golden years, to living life on your terms, and to the incredible adventures that await us. Let's raise a toast to retirement – a time to explore, prosper, and achieve our dreams. Happy retirement, my friend, and remember, the journey is just beginning.

A Note From the Author

Hey there, and congratulations on your retirement!

We hope this message finds you in high spirits and ready to embark on your retirement adventure, or maybe you've already begun your journey. Either way, we have a simple yet powerful request that can make a world of difference, not just for us but for countless others who are about to step into this exciting phase of life.

You see, we believe that retirement is a unique and transformative chapter filled with boundless possibilities, and we want to share the wealth of knowledge, inspiration, and insights that we've poured into our book on Retirement Activities: Embracing Life's New Chapter. But here's where we need your help.

Leaving a review for our book is not just about giving us a pat on the back (although that's always nice); it's about creating a ripple effect of positivity and guidance for others who are navigating their retirement journey. By sharing your thoughts and experiences through a review, you're not only helping us but also serving as a guiding light for those who are just starting out.

Let's take a moment to consider the power of helping others. Think back to a time when someone's advice or recommendation made a significant difference in your life. It might have been a friend's suggestion for a great restaurant, a colleague's tip on a life hack, or a neighbor's recommendation for the best gardening tools. Now, imagine being that guiding voice for someone who is about to begin developing their own retirement path. Your review can be that beacon of insight and support.

Leaving a review is your opportunity to deliver value to others during their retirement experience. Your words can provide clarity, encouragement, and inspiration to those who may have questions or concerns or simply seek a dose of motivation. Your review can be the guiding hand that helps someone embrace the possibilities of retirement with confidence and excitement.

So, why do we need your review? Well, it's not just about us—it's about building a community of retirees who share wisdom and support one another. Your review can help us reach more retirees, ensuring that they have access to the guidance and inspiration they need. It's about paying it forward, creating a network of retirees who uplift and empower each other.

Leaving a review is easy! Here's how you can do it:

- Visit the book's page on your preferred platform (Amazon, Goodreads, etc.).

- Scroll down to the "Customer Reviews" section.

- Click on the "Write a Customer Review" button.

- Share your honest thoughts, experiences, and any insights you gained from the book.

- Click "Submit" to post your review.

The impact of your review is immeasurable. By sharing your thoughts, you're not only helping us improve and reach more readers but also becoming part of a community that supports and guides one another through the vibrant journey of retirement.

So, what do you say? Will you be that guiding light for someone else's retirement journey? Will you help us build a community of retirees who uplift and inspire each other?

Leave a review today and be a part of something extraordinary. Together, we can make retirement a time of exploration, prosperity, and the fulfillment of dreams for everyone. Thank you for being a part of this incredible journey with us!

Lorie Eubank

REFERENCES

- *Breaking down 6 common retirement planning myths*
  https://www.ameriprise.com/financial-goals-priorities/retirement/shedding-light-on-the-myths-of-retirement

- *10 Life-Changing Benefits of Active Living for Seniors*
  https://www.holidayretirement.com/10-life-changing-benefits-of-active-living-for-seniors/

- *Budgeting for the 4 Phases of Retirement - Investopedia*
  https://www.investopedia.com/articles/personal-finance/110315/4-phases-retirement-and-how-budget-them.asp#:~:text=Write%20down%20and%20tally%20all,need%20to%20spend%20on%20healthcare.

- *Hobbies that Boost Mental Health in Retirement*
  https://anzmh.asn.au/blog/hobbies-that-boost-mental-health-in-retirement

- *Engaging in hobbies boosts mental well-being for seniors*
  https://www.news-medical.net/news/20230913/Enga

ging-in-hobbies-boosts-mental-well-being-for-seniors-s
tudy-finds.aspx

- *How to Budget for Hobbies in Retirement* https://www.53.com/content/fifth-third/en/financial-insights/personal/retirement-planning/how-to-budget-for-hobbies-in-retirement.html

- *Benefits of Traveling Later in Life* https://www.leisurecare.com/resources/benefits-senior-travel/

- *8 entrepreneurs over 60 who have started successful ...* https://enterpriseleague.com/blog/entrepreneurs-over-60/

- *Mindfulness Meditation for Seniors & Benefits | Mindworks* https://mindworks.org/blog/meditation-for-seniors/

- *5 of the Best Online Learning Platforms for Seniors (and . . .* https://www.helpcloud.com/blog/5-of-the-best-online-learning-platforms-for-seniors-and-why-each-is-awesome/

- *6 Brain Exercises For Seniors: Boost Your Cognition* https://www.forbes.com/health/healthy-aging/brain-exercises/

- *How Positive Thinking Can Help You Live Longer* https://www.verywellmind.com/positive-thinking-and-aging-2224134

- *The Importance of Physical Activity Exercise among Older* ... https://www.ncbi.nlm.nih.gov/pmc/articles/PMC6304477/

- *7 Low Impact Exercises for Older Adults to Stay Active* https://www.humangood.org/resources/senior-living-blog/low-impact-exercises-for-older-adults

- *Nutrition needs when you're over 65* https://www.betterhealth.vic.gov.au/health/healthyliving/Nutrition-needs-when-youre-over-65

- *Why It's Vital to Maintain a Schedule in Retirement* https://www.newretirement.com/retirement/the-secret-to-a-happy-retirement-a-schedule/

- *6 Scientifically-backed Benefits of Social Interactions for* . . . https://element3health.com/social-activity/6-scientifically-backed-benefits-of-social-interactions-for-seniors/

- *10 Senior Clubs to Join* https://money.usnews.com/money/retirement/aging/articles/senior-clubs-to-join

- *12 Benefits of Volunteering After Retirement* https://secondwindmovement.com/benefits-of-volunteering-after-retirement/

- *Why Family Relationships are Important for Seniors* https://seniornews.com/family-relationships-important-seniors/

- *Benefits of Traveling for Seniors - Cognitive Physical and* https://www.assistedvillas.com/benefits-of-traveling-for-seniors/

- *12 Budget Vacation Destinations for Seniors* https://blog.cheapism.com/best-travel-destinations-for-seniors-15235/

- *How to Plan for Travel in Retirement* https://www.investopedia.com/retirement/how-plan-travel-retirement/

- *Older Adults and Healthy Travel* https://wwwnc.cdc.gov/travel/page/senior-citizens

- *Creativity and art therapies to promote healthy aging* https://www.ncbi.nlm.nih.gov/pmc/articles/PMC9549330/

- *Be Artistic | Senior Services*

https://www.talgov.com/seniors/beartistic.aspx

- *Effects of Dancing on Cognition in Healthy Older Adults* https://www.ncbi.nlm.nih.gov/pmc/articles/PMC706 1925/

- *Lifetime Arts – National Leaders in Creative Aging Program ...* https://www.lifetimearts.org/

- *The 9 Best Computer Classes For Seniors To Learn ...* https://californiamobility.com/the-10-best-computer-classes-for-seniors-to-learn-the-basics/

- *5 of the Best Online Learning Platforms for Seniors (and* .   .   . https://www.helpcloud.com/blog/5-of-the-best-onlin e-learning-platforms-for-seniors-and-why-each-is-awes ome/

- *Older   Adults   and   Social   Media* https://www.pewresearch.org/internet/2010/08/27/o lder-adults-and-social-media/

- *The   Senior's   Guide   to   Online   Safety* https://connectsafely.org/seniors-guide-to-online-safet y/

- *Benefits of Hobbies for Older Adults - The Bristal Blog* https://blog.thebristal.com/benefits-of-hobbies-for-ol

der-adults

- *Healthy Aging Recipes* https://www.eatingwell.com/recipes/18053/lifestyle-diets/healthy-aging/

- *What Is the Evidence to Support the Use of Therapeutic* . . . https://www.ncbi.nlm.nih.gov/pmc/articles/PMC3372556/

- *7 DIY Home Improvement Ideas for Your Forever House* https://www.aarp.org/home-family/your-home/info-2021/diy-home-improvement-ideas.html

- *5 Retirement Planning Steps to Take* https://www.investopedia.com/articles/retirement/11/5-steps-to-retirement-plan.asp

- *Health care costs in retirement* https://www.usatoday.com/money/blueprint/retirement/healthcare-costs-in-retirement/

- *6 Low-Risk Investments With High Returns for Retirees* https://money.usnews.com/investing/investing-advice/articles/high-return-low-risk-investments-for-retirees

- *Estate Planning in Retirement | Key Components & ...* https://www.financestrategists.com/estate-planning-la

wyer/estate-planning-in-retirement/

- *Tips for Seniors on Meeting the Challenges of Downsizing* https://www.assuredassistedliving.com/tips-for-seniors-on-meeting-the-challenges-of-downsizing

- *10 Aging in Place Home Modifications for Seniors* https://www.homeadvisor.com/r/aging-in-place-home-modifications/

- *Cost Considerations of RV Living in Retirement* https://after50finances.com/home/cost-considerations-of-rv-living-in-retirement/

- *Top 10 Active Retirement Communities in the U.S.* https://www.investopedia.com/articles/retirement/082316/top-10-active-retirement-communities-us.asp

- *Making The Most Of An Encore Career* https://www.forbes.com/sites/jamiehopkins/2019/02/04/making-the-most-of-an-encore-career/

- *5 Benefits of Working After Retirement* https://benefits.com/retirement/working-after-retirement/

- *4 Steps To Finding Your Encore Career* https://www.beyonddiscoverycoaching.com/blog/4-st

eps-to-finding-your-encore-career

- *Work, Leisure, and Retirement | Gerontology - Oxford Academic* https://academic.oup.com/book/12561/chapter/162344662

- 70 retirement quotes that will resonate with any retiree https://www.southernliving.com/culture/retirement-quotes

- 'It was seen as an elderly white lady thing to do': meet the new generation of male knitters https://www.theguardian.com/lifeandstyle/2021/apr/10/it-was-seen-as-an-elderly-white-lady-thing-to-do-meet-the-new-generation-of-male-knitters